Contents

List of Contributors   v

Foreword   vi

1   The NHS research and development strategy   1
Simon Kirk

2   Morality and ethics of clinical and health services research   9
Antony J Franks

3   Challenging ignorance   19
Mark R Baker

4   Developing, disseminating and using research information   27
Simon Kirk

5   Taking advantage of the new environment for research and development   37
Anthony J Culyer

6   Health services research – a radical approach to cross the research and development divide?   51
Andrew F Long

7   Research and development in nursing and the professions allied to medicine   65
Rebecca Malby

8   Research in primary care settings and at the interface with secondary care   75
Alison Evans

9   Managing research and development   89
     Antony J Franks

10   Implementing the results of research and development
     in clinical and managerial practice   103
     Stephen Harrison

11   Future patterns   115
     Mark R Baker

Index   123

Research and Development for the NHS:
evidence, evaluation and effectiveness

Edited by

Mark Baker
Executive Medical Director, North Yorkshire Health Authority and
External Professor of Public Health, University of Leeds

and

Simon Kirk
Development Manager, North Yorkshire Health Authority

with a Foreword by

Donald Irvine
President, General Medical Council

RADCLIFFE MEDICAL PRESS
OXFORD AND NEW YORK

© 1996 Mark Baker and Simon Kirk

Radcliffe Medical Press Ltd
18 Marcham Road, Abingdon, Oxon OX14 1AA, UK

Radcliffe Medical Press, Inc.
141 Fifth Avenue, New York, NY 10010, USA

British Library Cataloguing in Publication Data

A catalogue record for this book is available from the British Library.

ISBN 1 85775 094 2

Library of Congress Cataloging-in-Publication Data

Research and development for the NHS: evidence, evaluation and effectiveness/edited by Mark R Baker and Simon Kirk.
    p. cm.
  Includes bibliographical references and index.
  ISBN 1-85775-094-2
  1. Medicine–Research–Great Britain–Management.   2. Medical care–Great Britain–Re-search–Management.   3. National Health Service (Great Britain) I. Baker, Mark R.   II. Kirk, Simon.
  [DNLM: 1. National Health Service (Great Britain).   2. Research–organization & adminis-tration–Great Britain.   3. Research–economics–Great Britain.   4. Planning Techniques.   5. State Medicine–Great Britain.   W 20.5 M235 1996]
  R854.G7M35   1996
  362.1'072041–dc20
  DNLM/DLC
  for Library of Congress   95-37786
                                                                                                    CIP

Typeset by Marksbury Multimedia Ltd, Midsomer Norton, Bath, Avon.
Printed and bound by Biddles Ltd, Guildford and King's Lynn

List of contributors

Mark R Baker Executive Medical Director, North Yorkshire Health Authority and External Professor of Public Health, University of Leeds. Formerly Yorkshire Regional Director of R&D

Simon Kirk Development Manager, North Yorkshire Health Authority. Formerly Yorkshire Regional R&D Information Manager

Anthony J Culyer Professor of Economics and Deputy Vice-Chancellor, University of York. Chair of the 1994 Task Force on R&D in the NHS

Alison Evans General Practitioner and Senior Lecturer in General Practice, Academic Unit of General Practice, University of Leeds

Antony J Franks Senior Lecturer in Public Health Medicine, Institute of Epidemiology and Health Services Research, University of Leeds and Honorary Consultant Neuropathologist, Leeds General Infirmary. Formerly a research manager with Yorkshire region

Stephen Harrison Reader in Health Policy and Politics, Nuffield Institute for Health, University of Leeds. Formerly a research manager with Yorkshire region

Andrew F Long Senior Lecturer, Health Systems Research, Nuffield Institute for Health, University of Leeds

Rebecca Malby Fellow of the King's Fund College, directing nursing leadership programmes. Previously Director of Nursing Practice at the Institute of Nursing, University of Leeds

Foreword

A deliberate attempt is being made to strengthen the research base of the National Health Service to improve the health of the community as well as caring for the needs of individual people. At the heart of this strategy is the belief that the NHS, to maintain excellence, has to nurture and sustain a capacity for new discovery, and for testing innovations and technologies of potential value. Linked with this is the belief that modern clinical practice has to become, more than ever, based on the best science available. Hence the interest in evidence-based medicine and clinical effectiveness in the search for better outcomes of care.

So, as never before, medical research is becoming everybody's business. Traditionally it has always been seen as the territory of academia, the interest of the universities and research organizations, standing closely alongside the business end of delivery of health care, but somehow not an intimate or indeed integral part of it. Today we are learning that this can no longer be so. Clinicians and managers who are not themselves researchers need to understand how research works, how they can use the results to the best advantage of patients, and in what ways they themselves can contribute to the strengthening of a research-based NHS. The interest does not stop there. We as citizens, and from time to time as patients, need also to become more aware of the role of research in modern health care. So, for ordinary clinicians, managers and patients, there is a need now for things which will help them understand this hitherto rarefied domain.

It is against this background that we have to see the government's ambitious programme of research and development in the NHS. Here is an important strategic initiative, without doubt one of the most significant of the health reforms.

Hence the importance of this book. It has simplification as its purpose, making difficult things seem straightforward. Written by a distinguished research and development team from Yorkshire, the chapters span all disciplines and describe the research and development programme in the NHS. The book succeeds in making this information more accessible and understandable to the wider constituency that I have described. The task is not an easy one. It is to the credit of the editors and authors that they have given us such a well-rounded text.

Donald Irvine
November 1995

1

The NHS research and development strategy

SIMON KIRK

The NHS and research

Health services operate on the basis of assumptions. These assumptions cover just about the entire range of the NHS, from its organization and management to its clinical content and the delivery of the resulting health care to the population. Assumptions, by their very nature, are inexplicit. They are the 'commonsense' currency in which we trade.

One such is that the NHS, or more particularly the clinical professions within it, 'do' research and, to a lesser extent, the other half of the research and development (R&D) equation – development. Like all commonsense notions, the assumption that the NHS has always included R&D is not entirely without foundation. The teaching hospitals and university-linked medical posts have always provided evidence of research output, whilst the other clinical professions have sought parity of esteem through similar intellectual endeavour. Meanwhile the Medical Research Council (MRC), alongside the other national research councils, has developed its empire of the basic biomedical sciences, ably assisted by the major medical research charities. Similarly, each of the Royal Colleges and most of the other bodies of professional representation has been more or less systematic in their individual pursuit of research and development goals. In addition, the Department of Health and its predecessors have a long standing tradition of reactive research funding and of central research commissioning. However, whilst patchwork quilts present interesting variation – not least in the unlikely combinations of bed fellows which result – failure to sew the different pieces together properly makes for a draughty bed.

This non-directed approach to research has produced a series of problems recognized for decades. Most recently, the House of Lords Select Committee on Science and Technology published its report *Priorities in Medical Research* which criticized the NHS for failing both to articulate its research needs and to attend to the problems of implementation.[1] With the possible exception of the defence industries, British science in all its many guises, has arguably suffered from the worst effects of laissez-faire attitudes. Consequently, and probably more importantly, the utilization of scientific evidence, near-scientific evidence and the otherwise justifiable, has been considerably poorer than it ought to have been. In the NHS context this laissez-faire approach has been significant in enabling continuing variations in professional practice and service organization and thus the health both of the population and individual patients.

Not another strategy

Forty three years after its inception, the NHS appointed its first national Director of Research and Development, Professor Michael Peckham. The agenda of his manifesto for coherence was in part identified and trailed by the Department of Health in the preceding year's publication *Taking Research Seriously*.[2] This report, commissioned to consider how to improve the use and dissemination of research, stated 'Overall, there is a need for a clear commitment to research, with resources provided for its dissemination and responsibility taken for its use'. The recommendations of the report were addressed to three specific audiences and are identified in Boxes 1.1–1.3: those responsible for the central commissioning of research, those responsible for managing it and those undertaking it. Although focused on the dissemination of research findings, the recommendations continue to make salutary reading.

Box 1.1: Policy Divisions *should*:

- commission research which is likely to be useful
- specify clearly the aims of individual studies
- clarify the products wanted from each study
- take an active interest in the research sponsored
- help to disseminate research findings
- consider the employment of specialist staff to advise on research
- commission focused reviews of existing research.

Box 1.2: Research Management *should*:

- develop a strategic approach to research management and use
- include a dissemination period in research contracts and provide resources for dissemination
- advise customers on research which may be useful
- assess researchers on their dissemination efforts
- establish a dissemination database.

Box 1.3: Researchers *should*:

- take principal responsibility for dissemination
- write time for dissemination into research plans and proposals
- complete specified reports on time
- ensure that publications are clearly targeted to specific audiences
- prepare attractive and accessible material
- produce and distribute summaries of their research
- disseminate research imaginatively and widely.

This (and other previously discarded) R&D challenges were taken up on the appointment of Professor Peckham and the April 1991 announcement of an R&D strategy for the NHS. His proposals for a strategic approach were first publicly delivered in June 1991 at the Royal College of Physicians and published in the *Lancet*.[3] He introduced his proposals thus:

> A research approach has not been brought to bear systematically on issues relating to the effectiveness of clinical practice, the dispersal and use of existing knowledge, the best use of human and other resources, and the contributions of medical interventions to the health status of individuals and the population. Neither has there been a systematic attempt to relate important health issues to the national effort in medical research ... The challenge now is to introduce a sensible mechanism for handling within the NHS the output of basic and applied research and to apply research methods to examine the content and delivery of health care. Such a mechanism is the only way of resisting the sometimes unreasonable and often unproven resource-consuming demands of lay, professional, and industrial pressure groups.

A clearer focus

Specific objectives were clarified and mechanisms identified with the publication of the 1991 strategic statement, *Research for Health*.[4] The three major objectives of which are, to make NHS decision-making research based; to provide the NHS with the capacity to identify problems appropriate for research; and to improve the relationship of the NHS with the science base as a whole, rather than solely with medical research.[5]

The scope of the new NHS R&D programme is deliberately broad, encompassing, in various degrees, every aspect from basic research to routine application (*see* Figure 1.1) and is consistent with the desire to improve overall co-ordination of health research (*see* Figure 1.2). Within the NHS, the strategy sought to improve the quality and appropriateness of

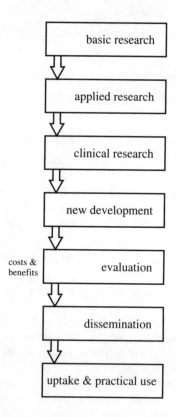

Figure 1.1 Basic research to routine application. (Adapted from *Research for Health* (1991) pp 4–5.)

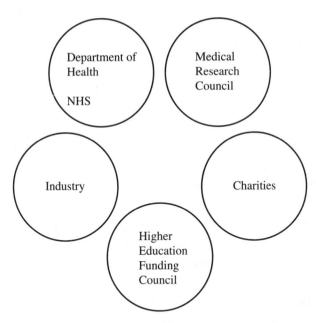

Figure 1.2 Co-ordination of health research. (Adapted from *Research for Health* (1991) p 3.)

research, the effectiveness of development, the stability of the R&D infrastructure, the consistency of R&D education and training (including that which enables a proper appreciation of R&D) and to secure the resources necessary for these tasks.

Within two years the Director of R&D was able to report an exciting degree of progress which had, over and above the specific tasks outlined, begun to impact on the consciousness of the NHS.[6] Such impact would not have been possible without an improved degree of clarity. A particularly necessary area of clarity has been achieved by defining what exactly constitutes NHS R&D (*see* Box 1.4).

Structures

The achievement and confirmation of such clarity is all the more remarkable given the current NHS cycle of change. The recently published Culyer Report[7] (discussed in more detail in Chapter 5) provides a detailed schema for the support of NHS R&D, comprising: a clear separation (and thus both accountability and guaranteed continuity in the internal market) for

---

Box 1.4: Definition of NHS R&D developed under the NHS R&D strategy with the advice of the Central Research and Development Committee

'All research and development whose direct costs are met with NHS funds should:

- be designed to provide **new knowledge** needed to improve the performance of the NHS in improving the health of the nation

- be designed so that findings will be of value to those in the NHS facing similar problems outside the particular locality or context of the problem i.e. be **generalizable**

- follow a clear, well defined **protocol**

- have had the protocol **peer reviewed**

- have obtained the approval, where needed, of the **Local Research Ethics Committee** and any other appropriate body

- have clearly defined arrangements for **project management**

- plan to report findings so that they are open to critical examination and accessible to all who could benefit from them – this will normally involve **publication**.'

(Reproduced from *Supporting Research and Development in the NHS* (the Culyer Report), 1994.)

R&D funding; a clear requirement for those undertaking R&D to justify their continuing receipt of support; and a guarantee of equal access to R&D funds for the primary and community care sectors alongside that of the acute sector.

In addition, the regional leadership which developed under the auspices of the first two editions of *Research for Health* has been confirmed despite the dissolution of the regional health authorities (RHAs) and the creation of NHS Executive (NHSE) Regional Offices (ROs). Although the exciting diversity of the early 'RHA years' may be somewhat reduced, consistency is to be ensured. The new regional structures have been indicated in a joint Department of Health and NHSE guide to R&D functions and responsibilities in the 'new' NHS,[8] designed to accompany the 1994 R&D plans of RHAs and clarify responsibility for the co-ordination and management of work within the R&D strategy.

The Department of Health's Director of Research and Development is a member of the NHS Executive Board and is supported by an NHS Executive Branch of the Department's R&D Division. Within the NHS

Executive, staff to support the R&D strategy are located in the headquarters and each regional office. In essence, at 'the centre' R&D is greater than the R&D strategy (including in particular the Department's long-standing centrally commissioned research programme, CCRP). Each of the regional offices will continue to include a Regional Director of R&D as part of the top management team, along with supporting staff, whose primary responsibilities relate to the R&D strategy and the continuing development of regional networks to ensure its success.

Identifying NHS requirements for R&D and oversight of strategic development are responsibilities of the Regional Committees and the Central R&D Committee (CRDC) plus its Advisory Groups. Funds in support of the R&D strategy will continue to be disbursed through a three-tiered mechanism. The strategic needs-led programme will continue as a mix of centrally and regionally co-ordinated programmes of R&D of national importance. (The Health Technology Assessment programme is one example of a centrally co-ordinated programme whilst an example of a regionally co-ordinated programme is that for Mental Health.) The needs-led programme will continue to commission R&D deemed worthy of support by regions, though not designated as priorities by the CRDC. In addition, Regional Peer Review Committees will manage responsive funding, on the basis of appropriateness to NHS needs and scientific merit. Liaison with other funders of research relevant to the NHS will continue as a central function.

Current variations in longer-term infrastructure support for research units and centres will be harmonized. Co-ordination of the various elements of NHS R&D funding (those described above plus the Department's CCRP and research commissioned by other branches of the Department and NHSE) will be similarly enhanced.

Where next?

The context and strategy described above do not imply that as the millennium approaches the NHS is miraculously set fair to make a fairy tale transition from chaos to a paradise of rationality. It was never thus (indeed, if that were the case the transition from RHAs to regional offices of the NHS Executive and the potential difficulties this presents to many facets of the R&D programme, would not have been a preferred option). However, there are hopeful signs, many of which are described in the following chapters: thoughtful and challenging contemporary contributions including reflections on research and development practices, as well as R&D enabling structures. None of the contributions in the following pages suggest that the problems of the NHS require solely technocratic solutions (whether clinical, managerial or structural) as each, in their own way, discuss and describe the likelihood of successful cultural solutions. Nevertheless, however much the service is willing to re-cast itself in the light of available evidence and coherently seek further evidence, we await similar signals of willingness from the political makers of macro-level policy.

References

1 House of Lords Select Committee on Science and Technology (1988) *Priorities in Medical Research*. HMSO, London.
2 Department of Health (1990) *Taking Research Seriously*. HMSO, London.
3 Peckham M (1991) Research and development for the National Health Service. *The Lancet*, **338**:367–71.
4 Peckham M (1991) *Research for Health*. Department of Health, London.
5 Smith R (1993) Filling the lacunae between research and practice: an interview with Michael Peckham. *British Medical Journal*, **307**:1403–7.
6 Peckham M (1993) *Research for Health*. Department of Health, London.
7 Culyer A (1994) *Supporting research and development in the NHS*. HMSO, London.
8 Department of Health and NHS Executive (1995) *Research and development in the new NHS: functions and responsibilities*. Department of Health, London and NHS Executive, Leeds.

2

Morality and ethics of clinical and health services research

ANTONY J FRANKS

Introduction

Ethics are the rules and principles which govern right conduct. Definitions of 'right conduct' are, however, conditional upon time, circumstance and individual; they shift and vary and may be impossible to reconcile in relation to a given problem.

The very complexity of human behaviour, and the range of socially-determined rules which influence it, is reflected in the fact that there is no clearly defined set of rules by which all actions can be judged, or decisions made on what is the right course to follow. Ethical theories are numerous although, in the context of medical practice, the two contrasting theories of utilitarianism and deontology are probably the most relevant. The former judges actions on the basis of the consequences, assessing moral rightness as that which maximizes the benefit (without necessarily specifying whose benefit); the latter holds that actions are morally right or wrong according to intrinsic parameters, usually determined by a set of underlying principles, which are independent of the consequences. The situation is difficult enough in cases where the act and its consequences relate to an individual but matters become even more complicated in the context of clinical research; here the act concerns the individual patient but the consequences relate both to that individual (in terms of clinical consequences of the action) and also to a broader group in terms of the knowledge gained.

There is, in fact, much common ground so that, irrespective of the theoretical basis, the same decision may be reached (albeit for different reasons). This chapter will not attempt to resolve these difficulties but instead will briefly outline some of the ethical principles which are relevant to clinical practice and attempt to relate them to the decisions involved in the planning and conduct of clinical research.

In allowing the medical profession a degree of licence in its use of treatments which have not been scientifically validated society expects there to be safeguards in the form of an overarching ethical framework. The possibility of permitting the introduction of only those new technologies whose efficacy is proved is now being raised. The intellectual drive to practice evidence-based medicine is receiving impetus from the need to meet growing demand with finite resources; this is a two-edged weapon since the quality of evidence may, on the one hand, support the reduction of unnecessarily complicated surgery (combined vaginal and abdominal hysterectomy when in many cases vaginal hysterectomy would be as good), yet on the other hand, make it difficult to resist the introduction of effective but expensive new therapies (cholesterol-lowering agents for hypercholesterolaemic patients after myocardial infarction).

Ethical scrutiny of all NHS-funded research is an absolute requirement. Most local research ethics committees are district based but many individual trusts also have committees overseeing any research dependent on access to, or intervention with, patients in their care. Whilst previously concerned with the ethics of a proposal there is a growing tendency to consider issues of design, confidentiality and cost to the host organization who may not be funding the research but who may have to bear additional costs as a result of the research.

Four basic ethical and moral principles should govern decisions in health care and research. These are autonomy, non-maleficence, beneficence and justice.

Autonomy

In exercising autonomy an individual is able to choose freely a course of action relating to himself or herself. An understanding of the action and its consequences is implied; even though this understanding may not be complete it should be sufficient for the purpose under consideration such as giving informed consent to participate in a trial (see below). This requires the provision and disclosure of information as well as recognition that individual patients have a right to their own views and beliefs when making a decision. In some forms of clinical trials (*see* Box 2.2) information is withheld from a participant about the therapy they are receiving; this fact does not reduce the obligation to disclose information relevant to the decision to participate.

Non-maleficence and beneficence

In exercising the first one should seek not to do harm, whereas the latter requires one to do good and prevent harm. These two are essentially complementary but the principle of beneficence may conflict with that of autonomy when it comes to 'knowing what is best' for an individual patient. Medical paternalism, which may be seen as an extreme expression of the principle of beneficence, is being increasingly challenged. It is not clear what, if any, ethical principle underlies the view that it is for society's good that individual patients participate in a clinical trial. The utilitarian view might hold that the maximum benefit will be obtained by this approach but violation of the principle of autonomy is almost inevitable in such a decision.

Justice

This embodies the principle of fairness in the distribution of resource or benefit. This should also apply in the question of patient selection for trials although uncertainties about the completeness of informed consent do raise the possibility that some groups (the less articulate perhaps) may be less likely to participate in randomized trials; if non-participants systematically differ from participants in some way relevant to outcome, a bias will be built into the study. Whilst not affecting the validity of intra-group comparisons such a study might be less generalizable to other groups.

Four rules derived from these principles should be considered to define ethical behaviour, or at least help to decide whether a course of action is ethical. They are veracity, privacy, confidentiality and fidelity (*see* Box 2.1). The last two are of most relevance in the context of research and development work.

Box 2.1: Ethical rules

Veracity – to tell the truth including disclosing the consequences of inaction

Privacy – limiting access to an individual

Confidentiality – limiting access to information about an individual

Fidelity – doing what one has promised (whether implicitly or explicitly)

Areas of ethical tension

There is an apparent tension between the deontological ethic (which includes the principle of beneficence) governing the relationship between the healer and the patient, (what is done should be with the explicit intent of improving the condition of the patient), and the ethic of utilitarianism invoked in decisions on priority and resource allocation (what is done should be determined by what will achieve the greatest good for the maximum number of people). The current social climate is one in which the concepts of utilitarianism are no longer entirely absent from the healer/patient relationship even if they do not overtly determine clinical decisions. In one sense the balance between these two ethical stances, and their influence on service provision is inextricably linked to the economic climate and decisions about resource distribution.

Against this background it is not surprising that research is seen as a means of clarification inasmuch as it may reduce uncertainty about whether an intervention works, even if it cannot decide whether it should be used. The increasing advocacy of evidence-based medicine reflects the desire not only to obtain the information (research) but to implement the findings in practice (development). The implementation of research results is not, however, free from ethical issues. In contrast to research where ethical review is the norm, no such controls operate when new interventions are implemented. The assumption that the introduction of an implementation is ethical if its efficacy is based on the evidence of ethical research is fallacious. As will be discussed below decisions have to be made about the applicability of research in a particular setting and such decisions must, in themselves, be determined by ethical principles.

Clinical trials

Ethical issues of informed consent

We have already seen that the principle of autonomy requires that patients are provided with sufficient information to reach a decision appropriate to their needs. In the context of a clinical trial such information may reduce the chances of an individual agreeing to participate (on the grounds that the choice of their treatment will be determined by chance or that one of the treatments may be less effective than the other). Such refusals may reduce the value of a trial; the ability of any trial to determine which of the treatments under test is more effective, is heavily dependent on there being sufficient numbers of participants. This has led to debate about the level of information which is necessary for consent to be truly said to be informed. One approach to this problem (a Zelen protocol[1]) involves the seeking of consent only from those patients who are allocated (randomly) the non-standard therapy; other participants are informed that they are involved in a trial but that they will receive exactly the same treatment as they would have done if the trial had not been in existence.

The effect of informed consent in reducing participation may be greater when one limb of the study is a placebo since participants may perceive (correctly) that they have a 50% chance of receiving an ineffective therapy (placebo) while there is a chance that the intervention under test is effective.

Box 2.2: Terminology and types of clinical trial

Uncontrolled – only patients receiving treatment are studied

Controlled – in addition to the group receiving treatment a second group of patients is studied who receive a standard treatment

Placebo-controlled – the group not receiving the treatment under study receive a substance which is believed to lack any therapeutic effect

Randomized – patients are randomly allocated to receive the treatment under study or the control treatment

Single-blind – the patient is kept unaware (blind) of the type of treatment they are receiving

Double-blind – the patients and the investigators are kept unaware of the treatments being administered

---

Design and conduct of clinical trials

In the quest for a knowledge-based health service the search for knowledge acquires a new imperative. Central to this search is the conduct of trials of appropriate size and design to provide answers to questions which will allow more effective health care. The activity is primarily conducted for societal benefit but is made up of treatments normally intended to be for the individual's benefit. While the study is specifically designed to maximize the chance of societal benefit (through knowledge) the individual's chance of benefit is randomized. In circumstances where informed consent includes the provision of information which will reduce participation to such a level that the results of a trial will be negated, who benefits? The Nuremberg code (written in the years immediately following the war crimes trials of World War II) holds that experiments should yield fruitful results for the good of society unprocurable by other means. A balance must be reached between societal and individual benefit and the risks to individual participants.

In establishing or conducting a randomized controlled trial it is implicit that an available therapy of known efficacy is to be compared with a therapy of unknown efficacy. In a randomized placebo-controlled trial a therapy of uncertain efficacy is compared with an agent of presumed zero efficacy. Only when it is not clear which therapy is better (new versus old, new versus none, established versus none) is such a trial ethical – there is said to be equipoise on the part of the researcher.

Biases in measurement and interpretation of outcomes are minimized by blinding investigators and patients to the nature of therapy. The potential ethical conflict between being responsible for the care of an individual patient whilst researching a treatment of unknown value is arguably diminished when the clinician is unaware of the nature of the treatment being given; however this may make it difficult to manage any complications of treatment and withdrawal from the trial conditions must be open to patients and doctors at any time.

Anonymity and confidentiality

These are particularly problematic given the number of people with legitimate access to information in the course of clinical treatment. It is especially a problem when an individual is identified for research purposes on the basis of their illness. They might then be approached to participate in research involving the collection of information or the collection of biological samples or the administration of a therapy under trial. There is no clear pattern as to who is responsible for giving permission for disclosure of information about a patient. Local research ethics committees express a range of opinions ranging from the need for specific permission for each case from the consultant in charge of that case, through to blanket permission for access to case-records for legitimate research purposes. Subsequent contact with the patient is not automatic and usually permission from their GP or the doctor in charge of their case would be sought.

Researchers can reasonably be held to be bound by the same rules of confidentiality (and thus non-disclosure to a third party) as those who have legitimate clinical access to the information. Anonymity is relevant to an interface with society in general (non-disclosure of information which would identify an individual patient) but arguably less so when, for example, the patient's name and other identifiers (address, date of birth) are the only link between disparate sources of data (such as police, ambulance and clinical records in cases of road accident). Such data must be linked by name in the first instance but can then be analysed and presented with no identifiers.

Termination of trials

If interim analyses are being performed (as opposed to waiting until all the data have been collected) the trial should be stopped once a clear result is apparent. Since it is not always obvious what constitutes a clear result rules should be built into the trial protocol defining the circumstances under which the trial should be stopped. From an ethical stand-point it would be unethical to continue a trial once it had become apparent that one form of treatment was more effective than the other. Unfortunately such stopping rules may prevent the acquisition of data relevant to the long term; a treatment may reduce short term mortality but over a longer period it may become apparent that it has no impact on eventual survival or morbidity among survivors. Once again the benefit to the individual appears to conflict with the potential benefit to society as a whole.

Although participation in trials may appear to constitute a potentially hazardous step for the individual patient there is evidence that patients who participate in trials do better, even when receiving the placebo, or less effective, treatment. This probably reflects the greater degree of monitoring, the adherence to protocol and the generally higher quality of care implicit in being under the care of a specialist.[2]

Experimentation, research or development?

When do trial results merit implementation? Meta-analysis, which combines the results from different studies, is one means of clarifying whether an intervention is efficacious or not; it may also show that the results still do not add up to a clear picture. Resources are also pertinent: a cheap, easily-implemented change is likely to be taken up more readily than one which has serious cost implications.

The concerns about the use of therapies which are, at best, of undetermined value or, at worst, experimental, have to be set against the remote possibility (or belief in such a possibility) that benefit will result for the individual patient. What matters from a research and development perspective is that once the decision to undertake a particular treatment has been made, the process should be guided by defined protocols, and its outcomes should be recorded so that the aggregate experience with the therapy can be assessed and, eventually, an evaluation undertaken as to its worth. Of course the most structured way to undertake this is in the context of a clinical trial where the likelihood of a valid evaluation of worth is maximized; the worst is to treat all cases differently or according to ill-defined principles.

One aim of clinical research is to define circumstances where a particular treatment will be beneficial so that others may reliably transfer the experience of one individual (or group) to their own practice. Herein lies one difficulty with the translation of the results of trials into clinical practice. Trials will, almost by definition, have strict criteria for entry to ensure that the groups to be compared differ as little as possible except for the treatments they are receiving. In real life patients do not come in convenient groups and their ages and clinical state often lie outside the limits set by a particular trial; for example the elderly, in whom the majority of heart attacks occur, are generally under-represented in trials for treatment for acute heart attack. The decision to apply the findings from a specific trial to a specific patient is therefore, in part, a matter of judgement, but what is often missing is the structured collection of data in the broader group which could address the question of applicability.

In addressing the question of which treatment is best for an individual patient the n-of-1 trial can be used. This is a study design which applies the principles of randomization of therapy and comparison of outcomes to a single patient. The treatments are used in a randomly determined sequence and the outcomes of each treatment period recorded, ideally by an observer blind to the treatment type. Since this approach is guided by the desire to discover the best therapy for an individual it is generally held that research ethics committee approval is not necessary if the therapies being compared are established or are considered efficacious on the basis of scientifically-valid trials. In these circumstances the research approach is applied to the treatment of an individual and the ethics which apply are those of medical practice rather than those of medical research.

Until the middle of this century much clinical experimentation was justified on the grounds that it resulted in increased knowledge and thus there was potential benefit to society as a whole. There has been a progressive move away from a philosophy of medical paternalism to one in which respect for patient autonomy has carried more weight.

Clinical research differs from clinical experimentation in that it is carried out following a predetermined protocol and has a defined end-point;

experimentation is a more speculative or *ad hoc* approach to the individual patient. As a consequence while the experimenter has the flexibility to adjust his/her actions in the light of circumstances the researcher is tied to a course of actions until a particular end-point is reached. Research studies will usually be designed to apply to a group of patients who have in common a particular disease or clinical condition, but each member of the group will be there by virtue of seeking care from a doctor. A research protocol may therefore place constraints on an individual clinician's course of action in regard to an individual patient; as discussed above research protocols must have clearly defined grounds for withdrawal (determined by the patient or the doctor).

Involvement in research may carry risks which have to be weighed against the potential benefit (to patient and society). Also relevant are the seriousness of the disease and the potential value of the knowledge gained. It is implicit in this decision-making process that the patient has given informed consent and that there are no alternative means of gaining the knowledge.

Conclusion

Clinical research and, to a lesser extent, health services research raise ethical issues which reflect the underlying ethical principles guiding decisions about care of individual patients. Difficulties arise when there is a conflict between the potential benefit to society from the knowledge which a particular piece of research may contribute and the risk to the individual patient from participating in such research. For these conflicts to be resolved it is essential that patients should only be asked to participate in well-designed, scientifically-valid research projects. Badly designed research is unethical since scientifically-invalid data are incapable of providing benefit and thus any calculation of risk versus benefit would be invalidated.

References

1 Anonymous editorial (1992) Zelen protocols. *The Lancet*, **339**:1574–5.
2 Stiller C (1992) Survival of patients in clinical trials and at specialist centres. In: Williams CJ (ed.) *Introducing new treatments for cancer: practical, ethical and legal problems*. Wiley, Chichester. pp 119–36.

Further reading

Anonymous editorial (1995) Your baby is in a trial. *The Lancet*, **345**:805–6. Places the issues of this chapter in the context of a current trial.

Beauchamp TL and Childress JF (1989) *Principles of biomedical ethics* (3rd edn). Oxford University Press, Oxford. A good general text which provides a more detailed consideration of ethical theory and practice.

CPMP working party on efficacy of medicinal products (1990) Good clinical practice for trials on medicinal products in the European Community. *Pharmacology & Toxicology*, **67**:361–72. Although specifically concerned with pharmaceutical trials most of the principles have wider applicability.

Naylor CD (1995) Grey zones of clinical practice: some limits to evidence-based medicine. *The Lancet* **345**:840–2. Addresses some of the practical difficulties with applying research results to everyday clinical practice.

3

Challenging ignorance

MARK R BAKER

A professional conspiracy?

It ought to be a matter of genuine concern – to patients, health professions, politicians and taxpayers – that there is little, and often no scientific basis for most of the health care which is delivered under the name of the National Health Service. Instead of high quality research, the factors which dictate the content of much clinical practice are subjective or even subliminal. Most of what we do, we do because we do it; history, tradition, obscure and often personal notions of professionalism and unsubstantiated opinion continue to dominate a high proportion of decision making in health care. This is true of both clinical and managerial processes in health care, the latter no less culpable than the former, and applies to all the key professions in the field.

This is not intended to be a one-sided criticism of the health professions or an accusation of conspiratorial Luddism. Indeed, although the deficiencies of previous practices have, for generations, been successfully perseverated by our clinging to the apprenticeship system of professional development and training, patients also prefer to depend on older 'remedies'. While the research effort in health is interested in collective outcomes, clinicians are concerned with what they see and who they care for, while patients are mainly interested in themselves and those like them. Each of these constituencies has a unique set of beliefs and values, such that a placebo effect can easily mask the objectively-measured ineffectiveness of a clinical treatment. This is why observed 'experience' often appears to conflict with research findings.

Many of the systematic attempts to improve practice manage to achieve little more than to legitimize current and ineffective practice. For example, the highly-valued and much promoted clinical guideline is often little more than ignorance dressed up as science if its content is not, as is usually the case, based on reliable research findings. The same is true of another favoured tool, the consensus conference, which often serves to guide recommended practice away from innovation and progress in favour of the *status quo*. These tools, and others like them, are useful in reducing the variance in clinical practice but not in achieving the change in culture which is often sought.

A deficiency of knowledge

Of all modern clinical practice in developed health care systems, it has been estimated (by Eddy amongst others) that only about 15% is of proven benefit. A similar proportion is of proven disbenefit or of no benefit, leaving a gaping hole of uncertainty about the value of health care. Even in the most robust and researched clinical database, such as the pregnancy and childbirth module of the Cochrane Collaboration, (*see* Chapter 4) more than one third of the aspects of practice reviewed are of uncertain value. Given the insecurity of diagnostic precision (a man-made tool to help man), the weaknesses of health service research methodology and the high costs of researching small benefits in health outcomes, it is probable that the optimum achievable goal of research-based practice will be little more than 50% (see Figure 3.1). Constraints notwithstanding, such an achievement would constitute a massive advance on current practice and would greatly enhance clinical effectiveness.

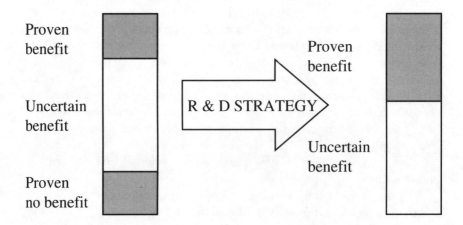

Figure 3.1 Shifting the spectrum of ignorance.

Establishing health services research

High quality, reliable health research can be difficult and costly to perform and, before the publication and resourcing of the *NHS Research and Development Strategy*, was unlikely to be relevant to the important issues of the day for the NHS itself. The NHS is a mainly reactive health system, meeting the expressed needs of the population for health care. For most of human history, the efficacy of care given by professional staff was taken for granted and not subject to question by peers or receivers. Such research as there was, focused on newly available treatments rather than older established therapies. The introduction of improved techniques of systematic review, including the meta-analysis of randomized controlled clinical trials, enabled and encouraged doubt to be cast on the perceived wisdom. Other analyses, such as descriptions of the variations in the practice of individuals, led to the realization that the health sciences are somewhat inexact. While variations in clinical practice might be tolerable, variance in outcome is not so; the infallibility of the professions is thus exposed as a myth. Some leading clinicians and professional leaders have now broken the traditional cartel of silence which formerly enshrouded any question of clinical fallibility.

Formal challenge to the decisions of health professionals is discouraged by the high social status of the health professions, the protectionism of the knowledge base – a core component of professionalization, the fact that the success of the clinician/client relationship relies to a large extent on trust in the former, and the widely-held view that, even in failure, members of the health professions act with positive intent for their patients.

The nature of the clinician/patient relationship also relies on the assumption that 'they must know what they are doing'. The somewhat unquestioning approach which this belief engenders is the opposite of that required to promote evidence-based health care. An assumption of ignorance places an unavoidable burden of proof of effectiveness on the provider of care (*see* Box 3.1).

The above describes a growing sensitivity of the health professions to the rising lobby for evidence-based health care. While there has been less than universal enthusiasm for this approach, at least in private, it does enjoy the high moral ground and a high degree of freedom from political dogma. It also potentially makes health decisions more accessible to patients, heralding the continuation and development of the slow revolution in the power structures of health care delivery. It may prove to be one of the great paradoxes of the turn of the millennium that professional authority and credibility will be sustained by openness rather than secrecy.

Box 3.1: Factors leading to a NHS R&D strategy

- House of Lords Select Committee on Science and Technology criticism of government funding and management of operational and public health research

- systematic reviews exposing the frailties of professional practice and espoused knowledge

- demonstration of inexplicable variations in clinical practice

- public and political intolerance of variations in outcome

- professional leaders espousal of research-based practice

- the rise of consumerism in health care.

Constructing a research and development strategy

To build successfully on this opportunity requires a systematic approach to asking the right research questions, commissioning and conducting the research to high-quality standards and delivering the products of the research in a form which is useable by purchasers and providers of health care and accessible to patients. These are the basic principles which comprise a strategy for research and development. A research strategy has a wide variety of stakeholders, each with their own views, interests and angle. The researchers, for example, like to do research which is of personal interest to them rather than the funder; they also, for practical reasons, prefer research which fits in well with their existing programmes. In consequence, research questions which are posed by researchers are unlikely to answer the questions of most interest and importance to the health service. Policy-makers, at government level, will tend to pose research questions which justify politically-acceptable, often pragmatic, solutions to short-term problems. Politicians do not normally commission research which sets out to question their own policies. Indeed, they are usually rather unenthusiastic about formal evaluation of any politically determined projects. Health purchasers and managers are concerned with setting priorities, rationing provision on any defensible grounds, currently favouring clinical effectiveness and cost effectiveness. Health care providers, including clinicians, like doing research which emerges from their own experiences, is easy to conduct in their own setting and is of personal interest to them. For many providers of health care, research relieves the monotony of everyday clinical practice. Sadly, it is exceptional for such research to be of general relevance or applicability and much of it is never published and therefore never shared.

Unless a situation of mutual interests of managers, clinicians and patients can be achieved, a research agenda which produces real benefits for all those stakeholders will not be forthcoming. Fragmented, self-seeking or self-justifying research priorities have characterized most health research throughout the period of rapid professional growth since the end of the Second World War left a vacuum in national and individual purpose. Health benefits, in the context of our nationalized health care system, must be counted in terms of better clinical outcomes for patients and better value for money in health services; commissioned research should also be subjected to return on investment analysis, the return expected being new evidence to support improved outcomes and/or better value (*see* Box 3.2).

Box 3.2: Stakeholders in health services research and their priorities

Management of high blood pressure

Stakeholder	Research interests
Researcher (medical school)	Further studies of the angiotensin converting gene
Researcher (health economics)	Cost benefits of the addition of a third drug to anti-hypertensive regimes
Clinician (teaching hospital)	Blood pressure control during haemodialysis
Clinician (general hospital)	Outpatient strategies for the control of high blood pressure
General practitioner	Improving patient compliance with hypotensive drugs
Health authority	Optimizing the results of hypotensive therapy in achieving the Health of the Nation targets
Patient	Minimizing the side effects of treatment
Complementary health interests	Non-pharmaceutical strategies for the control of high blood pressure

Harnessing enthusiasm

Many professional staff in the health service consider that they have a divine right to conduct research in their employers' time. In many cases however they possess neither the skills nor the networks for such research to be of value. The opportunity cost to the NHS of this personal research has never been calculated but may well be of the order of £100m. Under the new single funding stream for NHS research and development (*see* Chapter 5), these direct and opportunity costs must be calculated and declared.

Research which meets the standards and relevance to justify NHS investment will be based on a formal protocol which is reviewed by research and clinical or managerial peers, suitable for publication, is relevant to the NHS and, normally, reproducible in places other than that where the research is conducted (*see* Chapter 1, Box 1.4).

Assuming that we manage to ask the right questions and commission the research from capable teams who deliver meaningful products, there remains the unenviable challenge of managing and implementing change. Others address these issues in detail elsewhere (*see* Chapter 10).

Transmitting the evidence

The development of global communications systems, such as the Internet, has aroused excitement at the possibility of creating universal and instant accessibility to all useful knowledge. There are, unfortunately, a number of obstacles to the achievement of this Utopian outcome. First, the scope and scale of knowledge about treatments which is required by all practitioners to guarantee evidence-based health care, especially in general settings such as primary medical care, almost certainly exceeds the capacity of the human mind. Second, while electronic data transmission theoretically offers the immediate transfer of, and access to, the evidence required, in practice the volume of evidence will overwhelm the intellectual capacity of the user. Third, in the NHS, in both primary care and in hospital settings, clinicians' workloads are too high to enable the knowledge base to be interrogated for each individual patient. The Internet promises an overload of data not the delivery of usable information; a probable outcome is chaos.

What is required is a systematic interpretation of the avalanche of emerging evidence, of highly-varied quality, presented in a manner which adds value and is appropriate to the enquirer. A particular challenge is the presentation of clinical effectiveness evidence in a mode which is welcome and usable in primary care and in multi-agency community care settings.

'A paradox, a paradox, a most intriguing paradox'*

There remain many paradoxes in the drive towards evidence-based health care and implementation of the *NHS Research and Development Strategy* (*see* Box 3.3). Foremost amongst these is the issue of speed. Clinicians always have to deal with their patients' needs in the present tense. Increasingly, purchasers and managers are seeking evidence-based answers to pressing situations on which urgent decisions are required. However, if the evidence exists, it may take weeks or even months to assemble and analyse; if the necessary research has not yet been completed, the timescale may easily stretch into years. The process of priority setting for research attempts to overcome this problem by anticipating needs but, at local level, the circumstances are heroically unpredictable and many emergency purchasing decisions cannot be predicted in advance.

A second paradox is the tension which exists between new and old; control of the introduction of new technologies versus formal assessment of the value of existing ones; assessing technology or getting existing research findings into clinical practice. The professions are less threatened by the formal evaluation of new – and still scarce – technologies than by the possible exposure of the ineffectiveness of long-standing practice. Yet the greater benefits to managers, and often to patients too, comes from the slaughter of scared cows.

The third paradox is explained by the reactive nature of health care and the proactive goal of management. People who deliver health care are under an obligation to respond to the expressed needs of patients; purchasers on the other hand promote the morality of clinical effectiveness with a goal of disinvestment and withdrawal of services where ineffectiveness can be demonstrated. However, proof of ineffectiveness does not remove a patient's perceived need for care nor the clinician's desire and obligation to do something.

Finally, the natural competitiveness of doctors in particular, and the need to inject some excitement into mundane clinical practice, has led to a high value being placed upon clinical innovation. In the internal NHS

*From WS Gilbert

market which has existed, at least in name, since 1991, innovation is taken as an informal measure of clinical quality. In some ways, innovation is indeed an indication of intellectual aggression; in other ways, however, it is no more than unevaluated copying or differentiation. The logical product of evidence-based health care is a health service in which patients receive the same quality of care and can expect the same outcome regardless of where they live or where they receive their care. Where, then, is the place for innovation?

Box 3.3: The paradoxes of NHS R&D

Speed: Decision makers want the answers now but research takes time

Old versus new: New technologies are easier to restrict or promote but changes in older practices have greater health and cost impact

Reaction and proaction: Managers want to disinvest; clinicians 'must' respond to patients' presenting problems

W(h)ither innovation?   Individual innovation gives way to systematic sameness. Which offers most to patients?

4

Developing, disseminating and using research information

SIMON KIRK

Information overload

Consider this. There are estimated to be in excess of 10 000 health-related journals. (It is also estimated that 'proven' evidence-based knowledge can take up to ten years to find its way into standard medical textbooks.)

In short, the possibilities and opportunities are endless – from the average postgraduate library to 'surfing the Internet'; from the Resource Management Initiative (RMI) and Integrated Clinical Work Stations (ICWS) to data routinely used in the construction of contracts. The acronyms are confusing, the concepts often unclear, the data banks are massive and the flow of information seemingly endless. At the same time research, in all its myriad forms, continues apace adding more to the store.

Box 4.1: Defining problems

inform v. Inspire, imbue, (person, heart, thing, *with* feeling, principle, quality, etc.); impart its quality to, permeate; tell (person *of* or *about* or *on* thing or subject, etc.)

information n. Informing, telling; thing told, knowledge, (desired) items of knowledge, news, (*on, about*); -**retrieval**, tracing of information stored in books, computers, etc.

Concise Oxford Dictionary

Consider also the degree to which any NHS professional – clinical or managerial – is able to consider the possibilities and exploit the opportunities. Perhaps a glance through the relevant bit of the weekly 'trade press'? Doctors' in-trays piled high with *British Medical Journals*

(*BMJ*) and *Lancet*s; managers skimming the bite-sized chunks fashioned for the *Health Services Journal*; nurses doing the same with the *Nursing Times* and GPs casting a weary eye over something published with the support of a drug company. 'Special interests' or a firm specialty base may add another one or two titles to the monthly burden. Overall, it is not a particularly impressive hit rate from a possible 10 000.

The R&D aspiration

Let us assume then that, although our ability to discriminate between the sources on offer is to a large extent compromised, we are in a data and information-rich environment. Let us also consider that in spite of this richness, changes in practice seem more the result of water dripping on a stone than a comprehensive and coherent response to this overwhelming flood of knowledge. We should also acknowledge that no individual is a large enough vessel to contain the products of this flood, even if such an ability were considered desirable. Therefore, if we are serious in our desire to 'shift the paradigm' and turn the NHS into a research-conscious and implementation or development-oriented culture, we require a technology for irrigation.

Information, in a knowledge-based evaluative culture, is about implementation development – the 'D' of R&D.

Following on from the previous chapter, we can entertain the possibility of a shift from doing research simply because (like Mount Everest) it is there, to doing it because it needs to be done. This, in turn, holds the prospect of a somewhat slimmer body of evidence on which the NHS might immediately focus.

Managing knowledge: production, dissemination, implementation

Discussing information in an NHS context should always be preceded by a note of caution, best summed up in the phrase 'technology is the answer; now, what was the question?' or by David Berkowitz's observation that when you have a hammer, everything you see looks like a nail. A long history of apparently product-free but nonetheless expensive investments have been made in NHS information technology (IT). The sum total of all

Table 4.1: Defining solutions

Problem	Solution
data/information mountain	ease of access (retrieval)
developing research information (a sense of discrimination)	specific information products
disseminating research information (evidence-based knowledge)	access plus products
using, utilizing, implementing research information (cultural acceptance of products)	emphasize the 'D' of R&D

this endeavour can be encapsulated in the oft heard cry 'but the Korner data doesn't tell us anything!' (Or, 'it's OK, we've got Medline on CD-ROM'.)

Consequently, there are some simple ground rules (*see* Box 4.2) for those wishing to go beyond their weekly journals, and for those whose job it is to encourage other NHS staff in this direction.

Box 4.2: Managing information

- Libraries should not be just information stores
- Access to information should not be the sole preserve of those with special technical competence
- What was the question?
- Utilize robust products to achieve marginal gains (the cumulative effect of which will change everything)

Strategy

Librarians have, or should have, a range of skills which are more effectively employed identifying, accessing and compiling information than they are by date-stamping books for loan. Whatever the setting – medical, nursing or health authority – a systematic approach to harvesting information is required. The starting point is to know your resources and make the best of them.

Those who are technologically illiterate, or only partially so, should not be intimidated. The provision of information is not primarily an IT issue and even when it is, it is surprising how even the most Luddite can be won over by being able to get at what they want when they want it. One 'Effective Health Care' bulletin can have an infinitely more powerful cultural effect than ten failed Medline searches.

Priorities

What do you want to know and why?

To avoid getting bogged down (even the ablest IT-monger or librarian generally has only the one pair of hands) be clear about your information priorities – 'just because it's interesting/I'm interested' is not sufficient justification for the expenditure of organizational resources. Distinguishing organizational or corporate priorities from individual interest is a starting point, though the latter equally requires proper servicing. In this way at least the newly-published products of research can be fed to those most likely to take notice or even use them – the receipt of appropriate and timely information is one of the starting points for cultural change.

In the same way that technological literacy should not be a barrier to information consumption and application, neither should the lack of a personal research base inhibit the use of R&D information. Trust the authoritative statement, once the critical eye of experience and analytical competence, has been cast over it.

Utilization

Put a premium on evidence-based change: link audit activities to knowledge; reflect on the organizational research profile – don't repeat, or attempt the unfeasible (find out what others are doing and don't compete unnecessarily); co-operate with others for qualitatively and quantitatively bigger results.

Providers need increasingly to demonstrate not only their (relatively expensive) research competence but also their developmental inclinations. Purchasers will effectively be obliged to support the implementation of proven knowledge and will be equally obliged to refuse self-justificatory custom and practice. In short, research capacity is of less value to patients than the attitudes born of research awareness and a willingness to innovate on the basis of evidence.

NHS R&D information systems strategy

A structure has been placed around these issues, at least in a strategic R&D sense, by the national Director of Research and Development. His strategy document *Research for Health* (1991) committed the R&D programme to developing an information strategy to underpin the initiative. In particular it acknowledged the need to give support to the collation and analysis of research and committed central funding to that end. Both the Central Research and Development Committee and the regional R&D structures were obliged to advise on and implement 'R&D information systems for the NHS to co-ordinate research planning and ensure effective dissemination of results'.[1]

Two years later a successor document was published, indicating progress and forward plans. The consistent theme has been to develop information systems which respond to those who need to use information from R&D, 'particularly managers and health care professionals requiring well-validated evidence about different interventions' and those who need to use information about R&D, 'so that important topics can be comprehensively covered and unnecessary repetition avoided'.[2] These information systems (using the term 'system' in its broadest rather than just an IT sense) have grown from the Department of Health's original R&D Information Systems Strategy Study and the survey which produced the first pilot database. The result is illustrated in Figure 4.1.

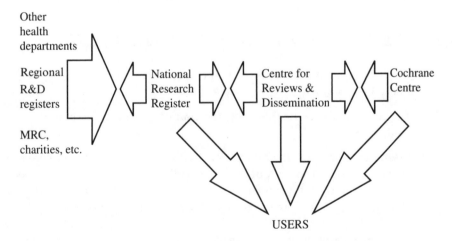

Figure 4.1 NHS R&D information. (Adapted from *Research for Health* (1993) p 20.)

National Research Register

1   A co-ordinated system of registers of research projects is being established by NHS regions which include all the projects they fund or manage.

2   A co-ordinating unit assembles these registers into a database, which will eventually interface with the registers of non-NHS research funders.

The Register is intended to result in improved access to information about R&D activity and findings, enabling better financial accountability, appropriateness and effectiveness and better research management, reporting, reviews and commissioning.

The UK Cochrane Centre

1   Produces systematic, up-to-date reviews of randomized controlled trials of health care interventions.

The work is organized largely by self-governing review groups. International enthusiasm has led to the creation of a number of Cochrane Centres around the world, whose work is collectively described as the Cochrane Collaboration. The Director of the UK Centre has stated that 'it will probably take a couple of decades to cover the past half century's evidence'.[3]

NHS Centre for Reviews and Dissemination (CRD)

1   Conducts or commissions systematic reviews of the results of good quality health research.

2   Maintains databases of these reviews and of economic evaluations of health care.

3   Disseminates the results of its own activities through the Effectiveness Matters update and through the Effective Health Care bulletins (produced jointly with the University of Leeds and the Royal College of Physicians) as well as the results of Cochrane reviews.

As with all new programmes, expectations have run high whilst tangible, usable products have been in relatively short supply. Nevertheless, the paucity of novelty should not obscure the fact that the NHS is still not able to offer conclusive proof that even the 'little' available is being implemented, to the detriment of the unnecessary, pointless or even dangerous. For example, a survey of the implementation of the key (and scientifically unassailable) recommendations of the first Cochrane database (itself a revised electronic-format version of the long-known publication *Effective Care in Pregnancy and Childbirth*) brought the following responses from some of those targeted as potential users: 'obstetrics is an art, not a science'; 'we're a teaching hospital so we don't need to know what everyone else does'; 'we've managed to avoid writing protocols so far'. The same researchers also pointed out that an editorial in the *BMJ* itself, ignored similar evidence-based recommendations.[4]

Everything, everyone, eventually

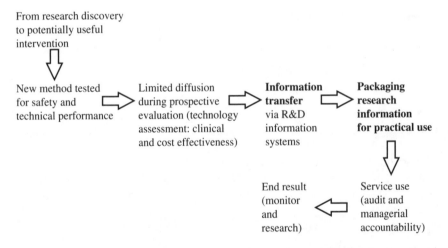

Figure 4.2 From research discovery to practical application. (Adapted from *Research for Health* (1993) p 23.)

The old adage that 'you can take a horse to water but you can't make it drink' would seem to encapsulate the NHS R&D paradox and is addressed more fully elsewhere in this book (*see* Chapter 10). Nevertheless, we should not be dissuaded by the apparent refusal, for it goes to the heart of illustrating both the problem and the solution. Whilst there has historically been no reason to do other than as taught (and confirmed through the experience of practice) little will change. Once alternatives are demonstrated to be both robust and beneficial, the hiding places become fewer. The premier product of high quality R&D information is not the inevitable improvement in planning, performance management and the avoidance of duplication. Nor is it solely an improvement in research performance. It is, above all else, transparency. For when information on best clinical and managerial practice is clearly and freely available (that is, what the results of research look like when translated to the daily grind), the clinical freedom to practice in any other manner becomes transparently untenable. Although this may apply in strict terms to less than say, five per cent of the sum of NHS activity, the iconoclastic potential of such a recognition is tremendous. The journey from opaque to transparent may never be completed, but the fact of it not being impossible reduces other explanations of why things are as they are, to the level of excuses.

Box 4.3: R&D information obligations

- Accessible formats
- Ownership through devolution
- Shared responsibility
- No excuses

The authoritative and accessible products of R&D information systems are powerful tools for recasting the NHS as a knowledge-based evaluative culture. The paradigm can be shifted and information can help us do it.

References

1 Peckham M (1991) *Research for Health*. Department of Health, London. p 8.
2 Peckham M (1993) *Research for Health*. Department of Health, London. p 20.
3 Chalmers I (1993) Making the most of the evidence. In: *Managing the Knowledge Base of Health Care*, R&D report 6133, Research and Development Department, British Library.
4 Peterson-Brown S and Wyatt JC (1993) Are clinicians interested in up-to-date reviews of effective care? *British Medical Journal*, **307**:1464.

Contacts

Bandolier – monthly newsletter on evidence-based healthcare
 R&D Directorate
 Anglia and Oxford RHA
 Old Road
 Headington
 Oxford OX3 7LF

Effective Health Care Bulletins
 c/o Nuffield Institute for Health
 71–75 Clarendon Road
 Leeds LS2 9PL

Evidence-Based Purchasing
 bi-monthly digest produced by the South and West RHA
 R&D Directorate
 Canynge Hall
 Whiteladies Road
 Bristol BS8 2PR

Information For The Management of Healthcare (*IFM Healthcare*)
 the Library Association Medical, Health and Welfare Libraries Group
 c/o Information Resource Centre Manager,
 Nuffield Institute for Health (address above)

NHS Centre for Reviews and Dissemination
 University of York,
 Heslington,
 York YO1 5DD

NHS Librarian
 Department of Health
 Skipton House
 80 London Road
 London SE1 6LW

NHS R&D Project Registers System
 The R&D Information Manager at the nearest Regional Health Authority
 (NHS Executive Regional Office from April 1996)

Purchasing Innovations Database
  The Kings Fund
  11–13 Cavendish Square
  London W1M 0AN

UK Clearing House on Health Outcomes
  Nuffield Institute for Health (address above)

UK Cochrane Centre
  Summertown Pavilion
  Middle Way
  Oxford OX2 7LG

5

Taking advantage of the new environment for research and development

ANTHONY J CULYER

Introduction

In broad terms, the flavour of the responses received by the *Task Force on R&D in the NHS*[1] in its consultation exercise can be summarized in five points: the system of support for R&D had 'just growed' (like Topsy) uncoordinated and in such a fashion that it was not clear either that the NHS's needs for R&D were being met (or even addressed) nor that the research community's needs for resources were being appropriately targeted where it mattered – at the work face; there was mounting evidence of conflict between the workings of the internal market and R&D; there was poor quality control and accountability; there was much confusion about what funding went where and to support what; and the system was not well-geared for the R&D of the future, especially in community settings for care and in non-medical health services research (HSR). The general rationale for the Task Force's recommendations has been discussed at some length elsewhere.[2] This chapter shall focus on how it is hoped people engaged in the R&D enterprise, whether as purchasers or providers of research, might respond.

The presenting symptoms (discussed at greater length elsewhere[1,3]) can be presented under three main headings: information, procedures and co-ordination; funding and service support; and costing and accountability. The principal points are contained in Boxes 5.1, 5.2 and 5.3.

Referring first to Box 5.1, there was much (expected) complaint about underfunding. As this was not a matter which the Task Force was asked to address, no comment was made on it. Moreover, to have done so might, given the heavy representation of the research community on the Task Force, and bearing in mind their likely prejudices on the subject, have brought about conclusions which could all too easily have been dismissed as self-interested and hence brought the whole of the Report

---

Box 5.1: Information, procedures, co-ordination

- general underfunding

- insufficient policy co-ordination between major funders

- shift of location of care and Cinderella status of R&D in community settings

- some arrangements only temporary (e.g. non-SIFTR, erstwhile London SHAs)

- disagreement about who should set R&D priorities (centre, region, district, institutions)

- threats to serendipitous, curiosity-driven and small scale R&D

- bureaucracy of the NHS R&D programme, poor announcements, poor feedback

- bias to medical R&D and to acute institutions

- bias to institutions rather than talented individuals

- threats to clinical trials (via ECRs – including tertiary referrals)

- uncooperative GPs (especially fundholders)

- Ethics Committees a problem in multi-centre R&D

---

into disrepute. But there was a unanimity about the other matters in Box 5.1. Several of the recommendations were aimed at securing better co-ordination through, for example, the new National Forum to get better overall co-ordination and the revamped Central R&D Committee (CRDC) which has now been revised both in respect of its membership and in the breadth of its terms of reference. All our recommendations contributed to the general aims of creating greater transparency, a broader sense of 'ownership' of R&D, and of widening access to NHS resources to the research community.

Box 5.2 indicates the main points emerging through the consultation exercise that concerned funding and service support: mechanisms had to be found that insulated the 'market' for R&D from the 'market' for patient care, not in the sense of building walls around each or making R&D remote from the NHS itself, but in the sense of ensuring that the way each 'market' operated did not act to the prejudice of the other. (Although the word 'market' has been put in inverted commas, being aware of the under-standable sensitivity of many to the connotations of the word, it is plain

---

Box 5.2: Funding and service support

- need to support existing centres of excellence
- need to develop centres of excellence in community settings (or in collaboration with community health professionals)
- cost of R&D inflated patient care prices and made R&D institutions uncompetitive in the internal market
- need for 'core' funding
- SIFTR too much of a general institutional subsidy (poor targeting from central perspective, money not getting down to researchers, e.g. research beds)

---

that there is a very special kind of market for R&D, whose characteristics, incidentally, imply quite clearly that its structure, got wrong, can do inestimable damage. One way of getting it wrong is to make inappropriate assumptions about the 'privateness' of R&D; another way of getting it wrong is to make inappropriate assumptions about the effectiveness of centralized administrative systems.) The main recommendations on this had to do with matters to be mentioned in connection with Box 5.3. The most dramatic recommendation made, however, was for the abolition of the research element in the Service Increment for Teaching and Research (SIFTR) and its absorption, along with all the other streams of NHS support that could be identified, into a unified funding stream which could be accessed for three kinds of support: support for programmes and projects, support for service costs of R&D (whoever funded it), and support for the R&D infrastructure which we termed 'facilities' support. Moreover, we were anxious to ensure that this funding stream was available to all potential R&D bidders (especially those researching into care in community settings), that it was allocated according to systematic and transparent criteria, and that quality controls were built in.

A further element in the diagnosis related to a keen shortness of research skills in some areas that were crucial for the success of the R&D programme of the NHS and of its information strategy: particularly in subjects like health economics and biomedical statistics (which were two mentioned in the Task Force's Report), nursing and the therapy professions and, not unrelated, in the research fields of community care, including general practice.

Box 5.3: Costing and accountability

- more accurate and standardized costing of R&D needed
- but not at cost of heavy bureaucracy
- extend National Project Register to include costs
- much R&D unevaluated (especially 'own account' R&D)
- move towards Higher Education Funding Council (HEFC) mode of quality assessment
- qualified support for peer-review

Box 5.3 contains the main points made about costing and accountability. On the costing side, we saw it as a necessary condition for R&D to flourish alongside the internal market that its funding did not prejudice the pricing policies of institutions delivering health care to health authorities and GPs (several recommendations fleshed the proposed mechanisms out). On the accountability side, we sought to achieve two aims: to ensure that funding to support R&D really went to support it (and not, for example, unrelated patient care) and that the R&D itself was subject to quality assessment (mainly via peer-review and periodic institutional quality assessment).

The general thrust of the recommendations can be described as 'enabling': they were intended to enable research individuals, groups and institutions to flourish, provided that they met minimal quality and effectiveness conditions, with minimal bureaucracy (though not none at all!), and in a way that supported the R&D needs of the NHS and provided the necessary NHS service support for the R&D of both NHS- (or Department of Health) sponsored projects and those sponsored by other bodies such as research councils or research charities. There were risks. One was that, in making the new funding stream clear as a levy on purchasers, they might signal their view of R&D (and also the short-term nature of their horizons) by systematically working over time to diminish the stream. Another is that the wholesale replacement of a largely automatic set of procedures for new ones that depend on pro-activity and initiative might find the research community as a whole wanting.

In the remainder of this chapter some of the main implications for some principal players in the R&D market place are suggested: specifically, researchers and research institutions, providers, and purchasers. In discussing these issues, some types of pro-activity that seem to be needed shall be proposed. The suggestions will be far from comprehensive but it is hoped, at least, to offer some beginnings upon which others may build.

Implications for researchers and research institutions

The Task Force wanted to see some shift away from a pattern of almost entirely providing support for institutions, like universities and teaching trusts, towards the support of individuals and teams whose past record, or future promise as seen by those best in a position to judge it, suggested that even a relatively free hand to pursue speculative lines of enquiry might be productive. Whether this opportunity is taken up will depend very much on the initiative of individuals.

Institutions will, in the future, no longer be able to rely on indiscriminate support via SIFTR. Instead they will have to mount claims based on reasoned cases for facilities support. The core of these cases is likely to relate to the provision of catalogues of overhead needs such as the need for animal houses, libraries, computing hardware and software, senior posts, research beds and the like. The extent to which facilities funding in the longer term will extend beyond these elements will, of course, depend on the persuasiveness of the cases being made. Such catalogues will need explanation and justification. Moreover, the justification need not be quantitative – the qualitative nature of a research community is of huge importance and some facilities support might be requested on grounds of, say, bringing biological scientists into more frequent research contact with clinical researchers. But at least of equal importance is likely to be the institutional context in which research is to be done: covering such matters as the institution's plans for R&D and its support, its general support in terms of resourcing from internal sources and its personnel (including promotion) policies, its R&D management arrangements, its R&D dissemination strategy, its arrangements for training and support of research staff, and the effectiveness of their networking with R&D-inclined health service personnel working in community settings. In addition, one would expect to see cases being made for partnerships, for example between the NHS, the Research Councils and the Funding Councils, in the funding of many overheads – a process that should be eased at the highest level by the new National Forum but which, at the institutional level, is one that should be started sooner rather than later.

Not all institutions are by any means adequate in the way in which they plan and manage their research programmes. In many of those in which R&D is most concentrated, the special needs of research workers on short-term contracts (who may even outnumber research and clinical staff on open contracts) have not been adequately catered for, with poorly-defined promotion procedures and matters such as the need for 'tiding over' funds for researchers between projects being left to departments and research units to manage as best they can with little central support or guidance. Contract researchers are also in grave danger of de-skilling over time, as some of the skills they acquired in graduate school are increasingly honed to perfection in the limited area of their research while others atrophy and newer methods, theories and techniques pass them by (this is particularly a danger where health services research (HSR), whether medical or social science in nature, takes place outside of and largely independently of teaching – especially graduate teaching – departments). They rarely have entitlement to the equivalent of 'sabbaticals' which could be used for retooling or developing some aspect of their research that is less driven by the needs of their external funders.

The location and organization of research is important too. It is unlikely that excellence in research can be built and sustained on applied research alone. It is essential for applied research to form a part of a larger (and wider) institutional (or departmental) portfolio of work which includes theoretical research, fundamental research with no specific 'customer' in mind outside the immediate academic peer group, and the more general work of parent disciplines. There are at least two reasons for taking this view. First, applied researchers, especially those whose work is almost always applied, need a more or less constant interaction with their less-applied colleagues so that new ideas developed within parent disciplines permeate the applied community and ensure that its work is really state-of-the-art and technically first rate. Second, this is a two-way flow: not only ought the fruits of fundamental research permeate the applied, but the questions arising in the context of applied research (for example, of methodology or of the applicability of a corpus of thought in an unusual field) should feed back into the more fundamental subjects and help determine both their research agendas and their teaching and training programmes. Within applied work, moreover, it is essential for the health of a research community that the priorities for research are not solely those of external sponsors: it is an essential leadership task to find room for applied work that addresses the particular curiosity-driven agendas of the researchers themselves or that is designed to test theories and the usefulness of concepts in applied areas other than those on which the researcher in question happens to have been working for an external R&D customer and sponsor.

Most HSR and much clinical research involves interdisciplinary collaboration. It is probably unwise to seek to prescribe the combinations of disciplines and set them, so to speak, in concrete. The rule ought to be to let the problems, or the characteristic problems of a field of research, determine the appropriate mix. Nor is it likely, given the immense complexity and technicality of the modern state of the disciplines comprising HSR, that the needs for multidisciplinary work are best met through attempts to create renaissance characters with skills traversing the entire gamut of specialist disciplines. That way lies amateurishness and mediocrity (the most casual trawl through early cost-effectiveness studies in the health field will reveal large numbers of studies fatally flawed through incompetent epidemiology or incompetent economics – occasionally both!). What is needed is teamwork, in which different members of research teams bring their own specialist skills to bear in the context of a shared research problem and where there is sufficient understanding of the potential contributions from disciplines other than one's own – and mutual respect – for the right kind of teams to be assembled and work well together. The disdainful attitudes still sometimes to be found, for example in fundamental science for medicine, or in medicine for social science, or amongst economists for other social sciences, indicate both closed minds and profound ignorance – indeed a philistinism of the most numbing (and useless) sort.

Arranging for an environment that encourages such things is by no means easy but it is surely a characteristic of the best places that serious attempts are made to address them. Not least in importance is the geography of an institution – the frequency of personal contact has been shown to fall rapidly with quite small increases in geographical distance, even within the same building.

A further implication for the research community lies in the importance of securing NHS allies, from purchasers, providers and at the political level. There is a major education job to be done if short-termism and a very narrow utilitarianism is not to be the dominant predisposition outside the research community. At one level there must, of course, be results and methods that can be seen to work, and probably early, in order to convince the 'Treasury mind' that R&D funding is well spent (and that more of it is needed). At another, the common penchant of some academics to berate the medical and nursing professions for their failure to adopt evidence-based practice is not one that is conducive to friendly relations, especially when those berated may have a powerful influence over the ultimate flow of funds. Genuine dialogue is essential, free of threats and free of any assumed superiority. This requires much more than merely the dissemination of R&D results. Academic research organizations need now to be developing links with local providers, which need not be teaching institutions, that will both contribute to the kind of 'technology transfer' implied by the aim of getting evidence-based practice more widely spread and to the development of local partnerships for further postgraduate training and local collaborative R&D. Most research institutions are located close to providers, whether hospital or community-based, which themselves have a number of research-active staff but who operate largely in a vacuum, with little regular contact with a research community, little support in the design stages of their R&D work, little collaborative help in the substantive phases of the work and a poorly-targeted dissemination strategy. Moreover, the internal support structures in trusts for much of this research (which the Task Force dubbed 'implicit') are poor, with much work often reliant on enthusiastic individuals funding some of their work out of their own pockets and in isolation from other colleagues within the institutions who are struggling on under similarly difficult circumstances.

Several higher education institutions have recently integrated, or shortly will be integrating, local colleges of health into their organization, and this too represents an opportunity for developing a research culture within organizations which have traditionally been heavily focused on training and practice. Again, local networking offers considerable potential.

Implications for providers

At the heart of the R&D strategy of the NHS lies its Information Strategy (*see* Chapter 4). A part of this is fairly conventional, covering such things as the Project Registers System and the encouragement of Royal Colleges to develop information systems on, say, emerging surgical technologies. But at least as important is the interfacing of the research and the practising communities. The Information Strategy is a crucial element of the drive for increasing health gain per unit of resource through the dissemination and uptake of evidence (that is, evidence from well-conducted R&D) to underpin evidence-based practice in medicine and the other health professions (including management). The different strategies of the Cochrane Centre in Oxford (now an international 'Collaboration') and the Centre for Reviews and Dissemination in York are mutually complementary but need to be complemented by further efforts. Mere dissemination (especially via the written word) has been shown to be insufficient. There need to be stronger and more personal alliances and partnerships forged between, on the one hand, those who are potential professional role models in hospitals and the community and, on the other, the research community. As indicated above, the research community needs appropriate leadership for this. But so does the practising community. Trusts can do a good deal to instil self-critical clinical practice by their staff but determined efforts to create systematic links between their own institutions and neighbouring research institutions are also needed. Collaboration in research is, of course, one such link. Others include the creation of well-crafted training courses of all kinds – well-crafted by virtue of early collaboration between institutions and individuals so that the product matches the needs and interests of the clients. Others might include the development of user-friendly databases of, say, cost-effectiveness studies, coupled with training in the art of judging what differentiates a good study from a bad one, and the art of judging the applicability of a result found for one set of places at a particular time in the local setting. Such skills are not normally acquired in medical or nursing school and, even if they were, they need periodic refreshment and revitalization. Senior trust managers (or one with a specific designation for the job) need to be sufficiently imaginative to be pro-active in these matters and to explore the possibilities with their local research institutions.

One of the reasons why the Task Force presented no estimates of the total funding for R&D in England was that there is no accounting system that currently encompasses it all (this despite the policy objective that 1.5% of NHS spending ought to go on R&D!). The major lacuna in the information is the R&D that goes on in trusts, without any formal external funding. Some of this is doubtless of poor quality (at any rate, unless it leads to a publication its quality goes unassessed) while some of it can be spectacularly good – many trusts are proud to have some, if only a few, consultants with international reputations established largely through what they have contributed to the literature. This implicit R&D is at grave risk in the internal market, for it raises costs and hence prices, without generating any compensating income stream unless purchasers are willing to bear the higher prices charged by institutions that have implicit R&D within them. A major and urgent task for trusts is to identify such costs as best they can and declare them, so that they can be protected. The Task Force recommended that initially these costs be protected unconditionally (once declared) and subsequently they be protected by formal claims on the single funding stream.

Each trust ought to have a senior (preferably clinical) person with an explicit title like 'Director of R&D'. The Director's task would be to identify the R&D going on in the institution, co-ordinate the work involved in declaring it to the R&D Division of the NHSE, and then develop a coherent strategy for own-account R&D that complemented R&D funded externally and that also complemented the institution's own post-graduate training arrangements. Such a person ought also to be responsible for liaising with the local research community outside the trust, with the Regional Director of R&D and the persons with R&D briefs in the trust's major purchasers.

The serious development of research strategies and appropriate internal support structures within trusts offers several attractive advantages. One is recruiting more able candidates to consultant and other posts and then retaining them, particularly if collaborative arrangements exist with local universities and research centres. These arrangements might take the form, for example, of college and senior common room memberships, joint appointments, joint research projects, participation in teaching programmes, or the award of honorary titles like senior lectureships or chairs. Some of these might be mainly symbolic; even sacramental: outward and visible signs of inward and spiritual states of grace, though nonetheless prestigious. But the substantive gain consists, of course, in the high-quality substantive work that such arrangements would make possible and in the seeding centres within the trusts that would be created through role models and demonstrable success in changing the culture of the provider in question. As already said, I doubt the effectiveness of hectoring and threatening lectures from 'outsiders' on clinicians' and nurses' practice, as distinct from the more specific but, in the long term more substantive approach, which enlists them as honoured partners in joint enterprises in which each contributor brings something essential to the success of the overall game and which actually yields tangible results in the form of research done and appropriately disseminated, lectures and conferences given and attended which would not otherwise have been possible, professional careers advanced and new, locally relevant, training mechanisms set up and running successfully.

Implications for purchasers

GPs, whether fundholders or not, are not typically strong on R&D nor networked into the research community. But some are. They now have their chance and a chance also to involve their colleagues in the nursing, caring and therapy professions. R&D in the community is probably best co-ordinated via the (admittedly too few) major R&D centres in universities, though there is nothing to prevent committed enthusiasts from creating local consortia of like-minded professionals, especially if they exploited whatever contacts they had with suitably-qualified individuals with relevant research skills. I suspect, however, that major progress in community-based R&D will come primarily from initiatives created in the universities.

Health authorities are another matter. Their role is crucial in a number of ways. First, they will definitely be on the Regional R&D Director's network and the more far-sighted of them will seek to exploit whatever advantages they can in order to improve the effectiveness of their purchasing by obtaining up-to-date information from the various databases, bulletins and other sources that are being created – and whose user-relevance could doubtless be much enhanced through a purchaser input at the design stage. Second, they will have their own epidemiological, public health, and possibly even economic, skills to promote the goal of a knowledge- or evidence-based NHS. Thirdly, they have an important role in encouraging their main contractors to adopt procedures that increase the use of effective clinical methods.

Networking with their local research institutions and facilitating technology transfer through the creation of relevant and user-friendly mediating arrangements ought to be high priorities for authorities. Authorities should also initiate their own R&D priority-setting processes, to inform regional and national R&D strategies. To designate a competent individual with a brief covering these activities seems the sensible way forward.

Health authorities, especially following integration with FHSAs, ought to attend not only to their own needs for R&D (and its results) to inform purchasing but also to enabling and encouraging the types of interactions discussed above between providers and research institutions. This is long-term work. It requires long-term partnerships (and less of an 'arm's length' relationship) between purchasers and providers. It might be facilitated in many cases by collaboration between purchasers in a consortium relationship that focused on R&D, dissemination and the development of a critical and evidence-based practice culture within providers of all kinds. Early examples of local success would be important, which implies identifying those institutions, specialties and individuals that appear to be most likely to bear early fruit, even at the cost of postponing R&D activity in topics that are actually regarded as more central from the purchaser's point of view. Changing a culture, even modestly, is something that cannot be done overnight or through heavy-handed tactics. The art must lie in a judicious combination of hard-headed appraisal and prioritization of the possibilities, selective support and bringing together of the relevant parties, and the creation or development of a generally congenial and attractive professional ethos.

Conclusions

The general tenor of the Task Force's Report has been described as 'enabling'. For it to work effectively demands the imaginative collaboration of all who want to participate in the R&D enterprise, whether as customers for R&D or as suppliers of it. For most, success at the local level will depend upon the active and energetic promotion of the types of principle that have been outlined by Regional Directors of R&D, and the cascading effects this should generate throughout the system. The more go-ahead purchasers and trusts have already identified individuals with explicit responsibilities for the development and support of the R&D function; others need to follow swiftly. An absolutely necessary element, which applies equally to research institutions, is the development of sound and constructive inter-institutional and inter-personal relationships. The emphasis has to be on mutual advantage; gains that accrue, or are perceived to accrue, disproportionately to one side only, cannot be lasting gains. Both the establishment of trusting relationships and the actual conduct of research from the pre-protocol stage to completion need time. Universities are well aware of the long leads and lags that sometimes occur in R&D. Purchasers and providers may well need educating in these realities.

A time of radical change can be intimidating, especially for those who traditionally feel themselves to be outside the R&D community or who feel threatened by the changes. But it also presents opportunities of two main kinds. One is the possibility of influencing the national, regional and (especially) the local environment before the arrangements firm up. The other is to gear up for the future in the reasonable belief that those most prepared to take advantage of the changes are likely to be those who will benefit most from it. It is suggested that there are potential gains for all three principal players: trusts, purchasers and researchers.

One thing is clear: there is no point in hearkening back to some mythical, halcyon past. The problems identified by the Task Force were real and were not going to vanish through evolution. There is no point in comparing today with things that happened a decade ago. But there is every point in comparing what might have been in five years time without the new arrangements heralded by the Task Force, with what can now happen. It seemed clear that disaster lay ahead, and not only because of the effects of the internal market for patient care but also because there was so much that was opaque, creaking, inappropriate, and simply unfair.

Whether the future anticipated here is actually one to be realized is largely down to the three players who have been addressed in this paper. Realizing the gains depends on imagination, initiative and 'can-do' spirits in all three types of institution. That they will fail to rise to the occasion is the biggest risk of all.

References

1 Task Force on R&D in the NHS (1994) *Supporting Research and Development in the NHS*. HMSO, London.
2 Culyer AJ (1995) Supporting research and development in the National Health Service. *Journal of the Royal College of Physicians of London*, **29**.
3 Culyer AJ (1994) Funding Research in the NHS. *Centre for Health Economics Discussion Paper 125*. University of York, York.

6

Health services research – a radical approach to cross the research and development divide?

ANDREW F LONG

A problem of definition

There has been an explosive, potentially overlapping and confusing use of terms in the area of health research. At the 43rd World Health Assembly, health research was defined as: '... the process for obtaining systematic knowledge and technology which can be used for the improvement of the health of individuals or groups. It provides the basic information on the state of health and disease of the population; it aims to develop tools to prevent and cure illness and mitigate its effects, and it attempts to devise better approaches to health care for the individual and the community'.[1]

A related concept advocated by the World Health Organization is that of *Health Systems Research* (HSR) and *Essential National Health Research* (ENHR) by the Evans Commission. HSR and ENHR is 'ultimately concerned with improving the health of the community, by enhancing the efficiency and effectiveness of the health system as an integral part of the overall process of socio-economic development'.[2]

HSR has however been more narrowly interpreted within the United Kingdom. Here its focus is perceived to lie on health services, their operation and modes of delivery, rather than the total health sector. Such an interpretation is reflected in the Medical Research Council's definition of HSR as '... the identification of the health care needs of the community and the study of the provision, effectiveness and use of the health service'.[3]

In part, this represents an attempt to broaden the focus of clinical research from bio-medical issues and an emphasis on randomized controlled trials, to health services-related issues.

To cast some light on this confusing use of terms, an alternative perspective is to classify the range of types of research by level and object of analysis.[4] Looking at the levels of analysis, research may be undertaken at the level of the individual or sub-individual or the group, community or population. In terms of the objects of analysis, the contrast can be made between conditions – the biological, psychological and social processes that constitute health – and responses of the society or its agents to health and disease. In this manner, a clear demarcation is evident between bio-medical and clinical research, where focus lies at the individual level, and epidemiological and health systems (or services) research, where interest lies at the population level (*see* Table 6.1).

Table 6.1: Typology of health research[4]

Level of analysis	Conditions as objects of analysis	Responses as objects of analysis
Individual and sub-individual	*Bio-medical research* basic biological processes; structure and function of the human body; pathological mechanisms	*Clinical research* efficacy of preventive, diagnostic and therapeutic procedures; natural history of the disease
Population	*Epidemiological research* frequency, distribution and determinants of health needs	*Health systems research* effectiveness, quality, and costs of services; development and distribution of resources for care

The aims of research and research utility

The aim of research is to provide information and evidence and thus to enhance the knowledge base for decision making. In the R&D process, research is concerned with acquiring knowledge and development with translating knowledge into action. However, the value of research is premised upon a rational model of decision making. As decision makers come to share common, better and more information, their opinions will begin to converge to identify the appropriate option or course of action. Such a model simplifies the nature of decision-making and the role of power of the varying stakeholders and politics within that context.

Even within a rational decision making model, for research findings to be used the research study must be perceived as valid and useful (*see* Box 6.1).

Box 6.1: Key criteria for research utility

Research should be:

relevant – a relevant topic area explored

timely – results available at an appropriate time to feed into decision making process

valid – done well and generate good quality data/results

credible – from the user's perspective

usable/feasible – recommendations for routine practice, and with the right level of detail

targeted dissemination – to the right people to implement/use the research findings.

From the researcher's perspective, the key issue centres around the validity of the study – has the study been done well and does it provide a contribution to knowledge? – disseminating the findings within a learned journal, rather than targeting them at key stakeholders. From the research user's perspective, timely research findings enhance their managerial utility especially if feasible recommendations for the application of the findings to routine practice are included. A key problem however is for the potential research user/manager to know that the research results exist. As Watt and Moir[5] observe: 'In order for research results to be useful, it is necessary for researchers to ask the right questions, and deliver the answers, or as near as it is possible to get to the "answers", at the right time and in an appropriate form.'

The core problem

While HSR is in vogue and seemingly has a high policy profile, at one level it represents little that is new. Research into the operation and delivery of health services has a long and distinguished history, even if its practitioners have tended to be health service researchers, not epidemiologists or clinical researchers. In addition, it is clearly not a discipline *per se*, but provides a melting pot, '... a space within which disciplines can meet, ideas be juxtaposed and research methods borrowed ...'.[6]

Most broadly, HSR provides an opportunity for research to be undertaken not just with other disciplines but across disciplines, or as

Rosenfield[7] describes it, to undertake transdisciplinary research. Within the HSR melting pot, a full discussion and analysis of a problem can be developed, drawing on ideas and perceptions of the nature and causes of the problem from the multiple perspectives and theoretical bases of the contributing disciplines. This requires a respect for the contribution other disciplines can make to solve the problem and an ability to listen to other perspectives.[8] Transdisciplinary research ought to move beyond inter- or multi-disciplinary research '... to a stage where disciplines can build on their distinct traditions and coalesce to become a new field of research',[7] that is, to integrate knowledge, paradigms and methodologies. HSR has just this potential.

HSR as a radical philosophy

At another level, HSR – particularly as advocated by WHO – is a radical departure from the traditional practice of research commissioning, execution and dissemination. WHO perceives HSR as providing a possible solution to the so-called 'application' or 'implementation gap' of getting research findings into routine practice. The core problem is the lack of involvement of decision makers in the research process.[9] This is particularly acute in the initial phases, in the identification and selection of the topic/problem for research. What is required is to involve key stakeholders – the research users who can make change happen – throughout the research process and critically in the dissemination of the findings. At the same time, managers and decision makers may have only limited experience or knowledge of research, or even strong opposing views as to its value. Managers need educating about research, its methods and value.

The problem of the application gap is by no means unique to managers. Indeed Tanenbaum[10] has queried the potential impact of the 'outcomes revolution', and by implication evidence more broadly, on clinical practice given the heuristic nature of clinical diagnosis and prognosis. This again points to the need for researchers to become more aware of the needs of research users. A classic example in the outcomes measurement field is the need within routine practice for simple, short and useful measures; yet researchers are developing longer instruments which will meet desirable psychometric properties (reliable, valid and responsive to change) but may be impractical to use within routine health care delivery.

The way forward is thus perceived in part as involving decision makers and managers in the research process, from problem identification, clarification of the nature and scope of the problem, and research design:

that is, as co-partners in the research protocol development process. In addition, researchers should take active steps to disseminate the results of their researches in a systematic and effective manner, targeted at key stakeholders who can facilitate the take-up of the research findings, and thus begin the change process.

But WHO's approach does not stop there. It advocates that HSR should involve the members of the community, together with other health workers, in research design – potentially in the undertaking of the research itself – and in disseminating the research findings. Research thus becomes empowering, for decision-makers and community members. Its aim is to change the conditions causing ill-health, exploring (more) appropriate responses to ill-health and increasing users' knowledge. The implicit philosophy of HSR is that research should assist in solving problems and that the end-product of research is action. Thus, by implication, HSR cannot be driven by the ethical principle of ensuring that the undertaking and results of research do no harm, but rather that HSR does some good and has a positive benefit to the community and research participants.

Available research methodologies

The current NHS R&D process is informed by the 'hierarchy of evidence' model (Box 6.2).

Box 6.2: The hierarchy of evidence model[11]

1   Evidence obtained from at least one properly designed ran-domized controlled trial.

2a Evidence obtained from well designed controlled trials without randomization.

2b Evidence obtained from well designed cohort or case-control analytical studies, preferably from more than one centre or research group.

2c Evidence from comparisons between times or places with or without the intervention. Dramatic results in uncontrolled experi-ments could be included in this section.

3   Opinions of respected authorities, based on clinical experience, descriptive studies or reports of expert committees.

The model is built around the notion of causation and, by implication, control of bias. At its pinnacle is evidence provided by at least one properly-conducted, randomized, controlled trial (level I) with descriptive studies such as the simple survey (level III) having less credibility as they provide only associational evidence.

The randomized controlled trial (RCT) gains its strength from the use of randomization as a way to avoid selection bias (chance dictates who is in the intervention and comparison group) and to control possible confounding variables (*see* Box 6.3).

Box 6.3: The randomized controlled trial model

Design

- random allocation to two or more groups
- one group exposed to 'intervention', the other to 'placebo' or 'standard' intervention
- before and after intervention measurement

Strengths

- no selection bias, but strict eligibility criteria reducing generalizability
- control of confounders
- limited information bias, if piloted instruments, standardized data collection, blinding of observer and unbiased end-point criteria

Weaknesses

- possible superficiality in questions/imposing researcher's frame of reference – for example, clinical rather than patient defined outcomes
- generalizability to routine practice
- ethics – is it ethical to withhold the 'best' treatment?

Efficiency

- expensive of time, money and people
- but, should lead to internally-valid study

Accordingly, provided information bias is minimized (for example, through piloting the data collection instrument and standardized data collection), the study will have high internal validity. That is, in relation to cause, there is high confidence that any effects observed are attributable to the intervention and not something else.

However, the RCT, like any other research method, is not without weaknesses. Firstly, randomizing patients to treatment groups may be neither ethically appropriate nor feasible. Secondly, even if randomization was possible, findings from a randomized controlled trial are restricted to the (narrow) population who meet the eligibility criteria for the original study, and the particular setting within which the study takes place. They thus have limited generalizability. The distinction in HSR between efficacy (does it work in this controlled setting?) and effectiveness (does it work in routine practice?) illustrates this issue.

Looking more broadly, causation is only one of several competing dimensions in deciding which is the most appropriate method for researching a particular issue. Another key dimension is that of generalizability. In contrast to the RCT, the findings of a randomly-selected, cross-sectional survey can be generalized almost automatically back to the source population. From the perspective of HSR the survey is an attractive method; its major limitation lies in its provision of associational evidence (*see* Box 6.4).

Box 6.4: The simple survey

Design
- (random) sample from a population
- systematic collection of data through interview or postal questionnaire
- one point/cut in time
- descriptive or explanatory focus

Strengths
- representative sample generalizable to the population
- lot of information collected in a short period of time
- depends on reliable and valid measurement
- statistical control of confounders

Weaknesses
- associational evidence
- possible superficiality in questions/imposing researcher's frame of reference
- limited control of confounders within the design stage

Efficiency
- cheap, quick

However, several authors have argued convincingly that this limitation is over-emphasized,[12] especially if explanatory (as opposed to descriptive) survey research is theory driven (not empiricist with consequent data dredging); theory-derived hypotheses can then be investigated through the use of sophisticated statistical modelling techniques such as causal modelling and logistic regression.[13]

The most problematic feature of the hierarchy of evidence model is its complete lack of acknowledgement of qualitative research methods. It is as if the only acceptable research methods were quantitative ones. Indeed, there is uncertainty within health care commissioning, amongst clinicians and policy makers about the value and credibility of qualitative methodology in health services research and thus the implementation and use of results from studies using this approach. There is also confusion over the term 'qualitative methods', which provides a loose description for a set of data collection methods – for example, focus group discussions, in-depth interviews and nominal group techniques – and a qualitative style of research, most particularly in the form of ethnography.

Qualitative research in essence entails seeing the world through another's eyes, the familiar looked at from the perspective of the stranger. The intention is 'to see the world as the other person does'. It is particularly valuable in 'opening up' a new field of study and where interest lies in understanding the meaning and interpretation of actions, decision making or organizations.[14] In the clinical context, qualitative methods provide a valuable approach to uncover patient perceptions of ill-health and possible causes and consequences, and more narrowly the nature and significance of side-effects of treatments and the issue of compliance. Contrary to misconception, qualitative research is not research into quality nor is it any less rigorous or objective than quantitative work.[15] Indeed, there is a clear commitment to make plain to the reader/user of the study 'how the study was done', together with a highly systematic process of data collection and analysis (see Box 6.5).

Research undertaken within the qualitative style moves through a number of stages. Within ethnography it is commonplace to separate a learning phase, a progressive focusing phase (focusing down on the problem area to be investigated), a hypothesis generation phase and theory building and testing phases. These phases are in many ways analogous to the different levels outlined within the hierarchy of quantitative evidence. A hierarchy of qualitative evidence can thus be drawn up, serving the aim of educating quantitative researchers and of enhancing the credibility of qualitative research for research users and decision makers in general. For example, at its pinnacle (level I evidence) would be theory and knowledge

---

Box 6.5: The general qualitative design

Philosophy

- seeing the world through another's eyes, the familiar looked at from the perspective of the stranger

Common forms

- ethnography
- data collection methods such as: in-depth interviews, focus group discussion, nominal group techniques, participant observation

Strengths

- development and manipulation of concepts
- aim to understand the meaning and interpretation of actors within particular situations, conditions and settings
- rigorous and systematic data collection and analysis
- interplay of data collection and analysis
- data are rich in description
- lay rather than expert definitions of concepts

Weaknesses

- reactivity (by the informant to the researcher)
- subjectivity (by the researcher – what to see, what is data, what it means, how to write it up)

Implications

- need for reflexive account – 'tell how the study was done'
- need for triangulation – multiple observations/points of observation

---

produced within the qualitative style which are generalizable to other settings by the very way in which the theory was generated (use of theoretical sampling, analytical induction and the comparative method in general). At its base would be the learning phase, comparable to a descriptive survey within the quantitative evidence model.

Within the context of HSR and health research more generally – and the credibility and take-up of research findings – it is critical to recognize and use the range of available research methods, both qualitative and quantitative,[16,8] choosing which to use for a particular problem by reference to the problem itself. Indeed, qualitative and quantitative methods can be used in combination, drawing on their comparative strengths and weaknesses and differing perspectives on a problem. Sole use of the hierarchy of (quantitative) evidence model – in research funding and in recognizing research studies worthy of implementation – can only result in the dominance of the RCT paradigm, the downgrading of the value and credibility of qualitative research, and an incomplete and misguided perspective on research methodology to the detriment of a deepened understanding of the causes and consequences of health and illness.

Evaluating HSR

It is evident from the above discussion that criteria for appraising a HSR study may need to be subtly different from other forms of health research. In particular, an evaluation of HSR should focus on its ability to influence policy, improve services, and ultimately lead to better health – a criterion of utility. Such utility draws on HSR's unique characteristics: its focus on priority problems, the multi-disciplinary and participatory nature of the research process (drawing in decision makers and community members) and research findings to lead to action.[17] At the same time as with any other research, HSR must be rigorous and scientifically credible.

A HSR project thus should not stop when answers have been found to the research questions posed, but should include an assessment of the decisions to be made based on the results of the study. In addition, drawing on the opportunity of the HSR melting point, a further criterion ought to be whether the problem is broadly defined (for example, in terms of range of possible causes) and the chosen method is the most appropriate (quantitative and/or qualitative).

Conclusion

In order to maximize the impact of research within decision making and to enhance rational decision making, HSR needs to be promoted in terms of the usefulness of the research process and findings to policy makers, managers and practitioners. Moreover, there needs to be greater participation by policy makers in HSR, to enhance their perceptions of the significance of research and to gain their involvement in the identification of research problems and thus their commitment to the use of the results of research. A dynamic relationship must be established between the policy, action and research sectors. Strengthening the linkages will increase the demand for and utilization of research results. Box 6.6 provides a summary of the issues, implications and potential output of HSR.

Box 6.6: Summary of the issues, implications and output of HSR

Issues

- A gap exists between research and practice, with many research results not being used – the so called 'application gap'. At least part of the problem has its roots in the lack of involvement of decision makers in the identification of the research problem and the lack of attention given by researchers to the dissemination of the findings of their studies.

- Information and action-oriented HSR is needed to assist health commissioning agencies to make choices in the pursuit of health gain.

- HSR must address priority problems identified by decision makers within the broader context of a national health strategy.

- Research is dominated by quantitative methods, with little credibility being given to qualitative approaches.

Implications

- Decision makers must be involved in the selection and identification of HSR problems, ensuring that the research undertaken is relevant to their practice-based needs.

- Researchers must give a high priority to the active and targeted dissemination of their research findings. The production of feasible recommendations must form one of the specific objectives of the research protocol.

- There is a need for education over the strengths and weaknesses of quantitative and qualitative research methods and the trade-offs between different designs.

Output

- Research relevant for action leading to an increased use of research findings – the fusion of R&D, rather than its separation into R and D.

- Increased credibility and use of appropriate methods in relation to the problem.

One question that remains is the extent to which HSR is able to separate itself from the bio-medical model, both in terms of causes and methods of research. The advocacy of HSR does not just represent a change of focus for research, but rather incorporates a different philosophy to research practice. Recognition of qualitative methods and their rigour taken together with the limited generalizability of the findings of RCTs to routine practice suggests the need for both a hierarchy of qualitative and quantitative models of evidence. Multiple gold standards exist, built on concepts of cause and generalizability.

As the debate on research into practice illustrates, it is often moot whether additional research is indeed needed. The 'problem' is not a lack of relevant information but a reluctance to modify practice, that is, to implement the results of research. If research evidence exists on what to do, further research is unnecessary; there is rather a need for a managerial commitment to act and use the existing research findings. Again, this is a core principle of HSR.

HSR has a synthetic role to play, encouraging trans-disciplinary research, the use of multiple methods to shed light on the problem and the use of qualitative and quantitative methods in combination. HSR aims to bridge the gap between research and practice, thus the key criterion of utility as part of its evaluation. Only time will tell whether HSR does indeed make a difference – will the potential contributory disciplines listen to or continue to shout at one another?

References

1 Davies AM (1991) The evolving science of health systems research. In: *From Research to Decision Making. Case Studies on the use of health systems research.* World Health Organization, Geneva.

2 Varkevisser CM, Pathmanathan I and Brownlee A (1991) *Designing and Conducting Health Systems Research Projects.* Health Systems Training Series, International Development Research Centre, Ottowa and World Health Organization, Geneva.

3 Clarke M and Kurinczuk J (1992) Health services research: a case of need or special pleading. *British Medical Journal,* **304:**1675–6.

4 Frenk J (1993) The new public health. *Annual Review of Public Health,* **14:**469–90.

5 Watt GCM and Moir ATB (1990) The Chief Scientist reports ... Strategy for health services research in Scotland. *Health Bulletin,* **48:**196–203.

6 Pope C (1992) What use is medical sociology to health services research? *Medical Sociology News*, **18**:25–7.

7 Rosenfield PL (1992) The potential of transdisciplinary research for sustaining and extending linkages between health and social sciences. *Social Science and Medicine*. **35**:1343–57.

8 Long AF and Eskin F (1995) The new public health: changing attitudes and practice. *Medical Principles and Practice*. Forthcoming.

9 Brownlee AT (1986) Applied research as a problem-solving tool: strengthening the interface between health management and research. *Journal of Health Administration Education*, **4**:31–43.

10 Tanenbaum SJ (1994) Knowing and acting in medical practice: the epistemiological politics of outcomes research. *Journal of Health Politics, Policy and Law*, **19**:27–44.

11 Canadian Task Force on the Periodic Health Examination (1979) The periodic health examination. *Canadian Medical Association Journal*, **121**:1139–254.

12 Marsh C (1982) *The Survey Method*. George Allen and Unwin, London.

13 Dean K (ed.) (1993) *Population Health Research*. Sage, London.

14 Fitzpatrick R and Boulton M (1994) Qualitative methods for assessing health care. *Quality in Health Care*, **3**:107–13.

15 Black N (1994) Why we need qualitative research. *Journal of Epidemiology and Community Health*, **48**:425–6.

16 Baum F (1995) Researching public health: behind the qualitative-quantitative methodological debate. *Social Science and Medicine*, **40**:459–68.

17 Batu AT (1991) Criteria for the appraisal of Health Systems Research. *Bridge*, **7**:1–2.

Further reading

Hunter DJ and Long AF (1993) Health Research. In: *Directory of Social Research Organizations in the United Kingdom* (eds Sykes W, Bulmer M and Schwerzel M). Mansell, London.

Lilford RJ and Harrison S (1994) Health services research – what it is, how to do it, and why it matters. *Health Services Management Research*, **7**:214–19.

7

Research and development in nursing and the professions allied to medicine

REBECCA MALBY

The announcement of a research and development strategy for the NHS was greeted by nurses and the professions allied to medicine (PAMs) with both expectation and some cynicism. These professional groups had called for a national strategic direction, particularly because of the difficulty they were experiencing in securing funding for the 'softer' areas of their clinical practice, and also because of their difficulty in developing a critical mass of research expertise. The scepticism set in as these professions perceived that the 'agenda' for the strategy appeared heavily weighted towards scientific positivist research methods, favoured by medicine, but not widely used in nursing and the PAMs.

The following year saw the launch of the *Strategy for Research in Nursing, Midwifery and Health Visiting*[1] as a response to the NHS strategy initiative. Its recommendations fell into four sections:

- structure and organization
- research education and training
- funding for research
- integrating research, development and practice.

Many of the points developed under those headings have been mirrored in the recommendations of the Task Force (*see* Chapter 5), particularly in relation to developing parity and equity of opportunity for funding, and in relation to building on and developing centres of excellence for R&D.

This chapter will explore some of the ways one region sought to address the difficulties facing individual nurses and PAMs, as well as institutions, in developing the R&D function; and explore some of the practical solutions that are emerging from the service, as well as some of the imperatives that are driving the R&D agenda for these professions.

R&D for nursing and PAMs in Yorkshire

In 1991 the then Yorkshire Health region undertook an audit of research activity among nurses and PAMs.[2] Eight hundred questionnaires led to an eventual response of 152. These contained 333 research projects. Analysis of the responses demonstrated the fragmented nature of research across the region and the pockets where progress was being made. There were many Trusts and health authorities that provided no response at all for nursing. There were others where a clinical specialty, such as radiography, had research as an integral part of departmental working. The majority research subject identified by respondents was quality of service (24.4%). The next largest groupings were education (12.6%) and effect of treatment (12%). The majority of this research was being carried out because it was a requirement of a course (39.7%), with 22.2% being self-initiated. The conclusions drawn from the audit were that research activity in the region was uncoordinated and not being disseminated. These findings demonstrated the difficulty that the region's nurses and PAMs were going to experience when faced with the opportunity afforded by a strategic approach to R&D. The response to the audit was described in *Developing the Research Resource in the Nursing and Therapy Professions*.[3] The regional role identified in this report is shown in Box 7.1.

Box 7.1: The Regional Health Authority *should*:

- identify a clear framework for the Region within which the resource can be maximally developed

- provide information on structural factors which support the development and utilization of the research resource

- provide a forum and network for nurses and therapists to stimulate debate and share research interests, reports, results and 'good practice'

- provide information on funding sources/availability.

These were matched by recommendations for service and education. The recommendations at a regional level manifested themselves in a number of ways, but the greatest impact was secured through the R&D network, that set the standard for investment in personnel to lead nursing and PAM's R&D within provider units. This approach to developing the research resource was matched by a concentration on initiating approaches to the 'D' end of R&D through the region's small grants for 'good practice' projects; the co-ordination and support for nursing and practice development units; and the regional learning network for clinical leaders. Moreover, the Nursing Directorate further emphasized its commitment to projects that linked into organizational strategy through its commitment to projects that tied into organizational strategy, via its management of the nursing and therapy audit allocation for the region.

This drive for an integrated approach to R&D, clinical audit and nursing strategy led to a picture that has been mirrored throughout the UK, of research and development support posts to the Trust Nurse Executive. It is likely that the trend was emerging differently in other regions, but all culminated in structures that emphasized practice development, with varying degrees of commitment to research. A new culture (particularly in nursing) of evaluation, quality standards and systems, dissemination of practice developments, and evidence-based practice was emerging with force.

Securing funding for nursing and PAMs

At the same time, the regional structure for R&D enabled nurses and therapists to secure funding in ways that had not previously been possible. The enthusiasm that nurses and PAMs displayed for regional funding was tempered by the difficult nature of R&D in these professions, highlighted above. One of the main difficulties faced by nursing applicants was that within the profession the term 'research' has been used to signify a whole range of activity and has become almost a colloquialism for small projects using elements of research methodology. In fact, these projects were usually about the implementation or evaluation of research-based practice, and are used to develop local ownership of particular practices. Whilst it would be possible to categorize some of these as replicative research, this was not the case in the majority.

This highlighted the need to concentrate on development of nursing and PAMs R&D alongside the regional funding mechanisms for R&D. Over the years, whilst funding committees bore the brunt of the fact that the percentage of nursing and PAMs applicants that secured funding was small in relation to the medical profession, the effort to develop the resource paid off. By 1994 research scholarships were being awarded primarily to nursing and PAMs applicants, and reflected the full range of these professions' research interests and methodologies. The initial fears that the R&D strategy would unduly favour medical sciences was proving false.

Another major block to research funding for nurses and PAMs was identified in the *Strategy for Research in Nursing, Midwifery and Health Visiting* – their exclusion from the Service Increment for Teaching and Research (SIFTR), which has provided a significant resource to medical research within Trusts. The Task Force report[4] sweeps away this historic inequality, with considerable benefit to the nursing and PAMs professions. The emphasis on networks and enabling in the report sits comfortably with the way that R&D has been developing within the professions. However, there is still a considerable way to go within Trusts if they are to travel in this visionary direction. In Trusts, medicine, along with a positive approach to research, still dominates. The cultural change that will allow research methods favoured by nurses and PAMs to be judged on a par with clinical trials, has still to take place at a local level.

Developing a strategic approach within Trusts

Many Trusts are still grappling with the notion that they should be supporting an essentially individualistic, and potentially professionally driven approach to local R&D. Moreover, they remain uneasy about anything that has a flavour of being 'centrally driven'. The Task Force report will find its enemies and friends amongst all sections of the NHS community! A number of ways into the problems are emerging. The trend mirrors that of clinical audit, in that most Trusts have taken a uni-disciplinary approach (or have put nursing and the PAMs under one umbrella, separate from the doctors) and are now moving towards a cross service and professions approach.

Nursing and PAMs managers are having to develop their confidence, as with audit, about their usefulness, credibility and function at the strategic table. Some Trusts have found it beneficial to develop a nursing R&D strategy that focuses on developing research expertise within a few specific areas related to patient need, e.g. tissue viability or infection control. In doing so, departments have concentrated their efforts around the leadership of individuals with the knowledge and expertise within the Trust to deliver research – incorporating that individuality into a corporate culture. The nursing department of the United Leeds Teaching Hospitals Trust has used this focus as a springboard for the development of national guidelines in pressure sore prevention and management. It has thus established itself as a centre of excellence and as a resource, through its research, to nursing on a national basis. This complements the strategic direction of the Trust and puts nursing on a footing with medicine in a traditionally doctor-dominated environment (at least in terms of research funding). This platform has led to greater integration of the profession within the Trust in developing the Trust-wide R&D strategy.

However Trusts go about developing their strategic approach they have to address one fundamental issue – the difficulty in getting nurses to respond to change. MacGuire[5] states that the three reasons for the 'supposed failure of nurses to respond to change, that nurses do not know about research findings, that there is an absence of relevant research to validate changes in practice and that there is a lack of synthesis of new research findings in a form appropriate for practitioner use, are themselves not well supported by research'. She suggests that an 'alternative view, for which there is considerable evidence ... is that change is found to be disruptive and is resisted by most people'.

This is a view supported by many nurses within Trusts and explains why the emphasis of R&D posts within nursing departments is on the 'D' of R&D. The posts concentrate on networking, change management and facilitation. This is in stark contrast to much of the R&D structure on a macro level, which has been about developing information sources. However, it does provide the complement that will make the R&D strategy workable locally.

Box 7.2: Characteristics of a supportive organizational culture

- flexibility in teaching, administrative and/or clinical assignments so that time for research is possible

- need for time to be used for such activities as thinking about researchable questions, library searches, discussion with colleagues, writing up the design, carrying out the study

- a system of formal rewards and recognition and research involvement such as promotion, salary and opportunities for travel

- an informal reward system within the organization, i.e. peers are supportive of active (nurse) researchers' involvement and productivity in research

- research productivity or recognition for achievement in research is shown through numbers of grants obtained, papers presented, manuscripts published

- sufficient (nurse) researchers in the organization to act as a critical mass for the development of research

- provision of educational programmes for the preparation of teachers and consultants in nursing research

- participation of nurse researchers in multi-disciplinary research projects

The International Congress of Nurses[6] has identified and developed the characteristics of an organization with a culture supportive of nursing research (*see* Box 7.2).

Box 7.3 indicates a number of models for supporting research and development, which were described in *Developing the Research Resource in the Nursing and Therapy Professions*.[3]

Box 7.3: Models for supporting research and development

The Implementation Model – where work progresses mainly through committee, in relation to the priorities of the lead officer

The Nursing Development Unit Model – where work progresses through the NDU with a practice focus and dissemination by role modelling

The Open Access Model – where work progress is based on staff concerns to sustain a questioning approach and innovation

---

Trust strategies are increasingly incorporating the initiation of links with academic centres. This is demonstrated by the dramatic increase in the number of University Chairs in Nursing, often sponsored by Trusts. However, the number of vacancies is not necessarily representative of the number of appropriate candidates for such posts. There is a lead time between investment in nursing and PAMs research infrastructure and the ability of these professions to deliver a return on that investment in terms of leaders in nursing and PAMs research. This resembles the chicken and the egg situation. There is a view that nurse executives of the future will be joint appointments with academic centres. This seems to be a change in direction from the drive to become a corporate player with an interest in nursing.

Priorities for nursing and PAMs research

As the tide of consumerism swells and develops momentum, then the 'softer' issues that patients find important in their care are beginning to emerge as important questions for research. Patient involvement in focus groups, forums and participation in needs assessment is beginning to highlight the things that they find important, namely comfort, information, nurturing, compassion and communication between professionals. All ways of organizing care to put the patient at the centre. Approaches to research that attempt to understand the user's perspective, i.e. phenomenological studies, will be exactly the approaches required for the modern day health service. Moreover, the importance of the context in which treatment and care takes place, which is becoming apparent as we begin to investigate why patients have different experiences of care in different settings, is captured and put into a cultural perspective using ethnographic approaches.

An approach that is particularly popular is grounded theory,[7] probably because it uses the actual experience captured by the data, to discover theory. This can be seen as the epitome of practice driving theory. All these approaches have been used in nursing since the 1960s. The challenge is to attain credibility for these methods within the wider health research community. The reality is that the current health care agenda (effectiveness, development, partnerships, consumer-driven care, understanding staff behaviour) favours the methods on which nurses and PAMs have cut their research teeth.

Thus the priorities for the health services favour the methodologies and subject interests of nurses and PAMs. The challenge now is to make that agenda a reality by developing national and local priorities for nursing and PAMs research. Whatever the priority there is still much success to be had from piggy-backing nursing and PAMs research onto medical research, using the nursing and therapy interest as a different dynamic to developing a research portfolio that captures all the patient's experience.

The overriding priority in terms of the R&D agenda must still be the need to convert research findings into effective treatment and care. The nursing research agenda must seek to demonstrate that scientific approaches in isolation do not capture the complete picture and cannot therefore be the sole drivers of the 'best practice' agenda of guidelines and protocols. The missing link in the chain from physiological evidence to the reality of human behaviour has yet to be grasped and appreciated at all levels of the R&D strategy. Nursing particularly attempts to balance the implementation of measures demonstrated to improve health with a sensitivity and regard for the impact of patient beliefs, attitude, self-perception and awareness, cultural and spiritual experience, and personal responsibilities, as well as the impact of the treatment and care environment coupled with the individuals' willingness and ability to learn. This is not to decry the necessity for research into the scientific base of nursing, rather to demonstrate that both art and science have their place in modern nursing and should thus have their places when developing priorities within an R&D strategy.

Nursing and PAMs R&D within primary care

Perhaps the area that requires the most rapid growth in terms of R&D investment for these professions, is primary care. The development of primary care-led purchasing and the move towards case management and integrated practice teams offers a wealth of opportunity for health services research. As nurses in particular move to take up key roles in these developing organizations, as clinical leaders, practice managers, case managers or project managers, they will be influential in setting and supporting the R&D agenda. Whilst the Task Force report[4] recognized the dangers of isolation and under-development in community settings, networking and the development of research priorities and expertise across such diversity and isolation will provide a tremendous challenge. For nurses and PAMs this is particularly emphasized by the lack of professional structures to support them within primary care settings. Many solutions are being developed but there is no established model that can advance nursing and PAMs research within these settings. This could be the perfect challenge for academic institutions.

Conclusion

Nursing and PAMs have come a long way since 1991, and have much further to go. The development of a broader-based research community for nursing, that encompasses successfully both the art and science of nursing whilst remaining sensitive to health service requirements, is essential. Even more essential is the integration of nursing and PAMs research, on an equal footing, into the R&D strategies of Trusts; and a career ladder for individuals within these professions that wish to remain closely involved with the R&D agenda. The key to success for these professions has to be in:

- developing local uni-disciplinary confidence before launching into a multi-disciplinary strategy

- recognizing the need to build on the interests and strengths of individuals

- marketing the relevance of nursing and PAMs research methodologies to current health services research priorities

- making the most of the funding opportunities which are being opened up

- making the most of developments in primary care to initiate R&D

- recognizing the power of developing centres of excellence for a range of health service developments.

The opportunities for nursing and PAMs are better than they have ever been, it is now up to them to demonstrate their fitness to deliver.

References

1 Department of Health (1992) *Report of the Taskforce on the Strategy for Research in Nursing, Midwifery and Health Visiting*. Research and Development Division, NHS Executive, Leeds.
2 Yorkshire Regional Health Authority (1991) *A report of an audit of research activity of nurses and professions allied to medicine*. Yorkshire Regional Health Authority.
3 Hamer S (ed.) (1992) *Developing the Research Resource in the Nursing and Therapy Professions*. Yorkshire Regional Health Authority.
4 Task Force on R&D in the NHS (1994) *Supporting Research and Development in the NHS*. HMSO, London.
5 MacGuire J (1990) Putting nursing research findings into practice: research utilization as an aspect of the management of change. *Journal of Advanced Nursing*, **15**:615.
6 International Congress of Nurses (1985) *Proceedings of Assembly*.
7 Glaser BG and Strauss AL (1967) *The discovery of grounded theory: strategies for qualitative research*. Aldine Publishing Company, Chicago.

Further reading

Armitage S (1990) Research utilization in practice. *Nurse Education Today*, **10**:10–15.
Buckeldee J and McMahon R (eds) (1994) *The research experience in nursing*. Chapman and Hall, London.
Field PA and Morse J (1985) *Nursing research, the application of qualitative approaches*. Chapman and Hall, London.
Lelean SR and Clarke M (1990) Research resource development in the United Kingdom. *International Journal of Nursing Studies*, **27**:123–38.

8

Research in primary care settings and at the interface with secondary care

ALISON EVANS

The term primary care strictly applies to all health workers who provide a first point of contact to the public. As research in nursing and the professions allied to medicine was dealt with previously, this chapter concentrates on primary *medical* care, which is mainly provided by general practice and its associated primary health care teams. The primary care provided by community clinics, e.g. in family planning and child surveillance, is increasingly being taken over by general practice-based teams. Primary medical care is also delivered by hospital departments of Accident and Emergency and Genito-urinary Medicine but structure and funding of research in those departments is largely the same as in secondary care.

The interface between primary and secondary care used to be clear-cut, with general practitioners handing over patient care to consultants. Shared care, e.g. in diabetes, open access for GPs to services previously restricted to secondary care, e.g. exercise electrocardiography and endoscopy, earlier discharge following surgery, and consultant out-reach clinics, are among the developments that have blurred the boundaries of primary and secondary care.

This chapter attempts to put primary care and interface research into context. It outlines the need for research in these areas, the problems both of doing the research and of putting research knowledge into practice, and some of the ways that these problems are being, or might be, tackled.

Background

Traditionally, research in general practice has been carried out by a few exceptional individuals. Prior to the foundation of the Royal College of General Practitioners (RCGP) in 1952 there was little in the way of support or networking for general practice researchers. The lone GP researcher had access only to his own small practice population, and probably little time or funding to carry out research. In contrast, time for research was built in to hospital senior registrar posts,[1] where there was easier access to a larger population of patients. In addition, most research funding went (and still does go) to hospital-based research. Despite the fact that this hospital-based research was carried out on highly selected patients, the findings were routinely extrapolated to the general population seen in primary care. It would not be surprising if primary care workers rejected 'evidence-based practice' based on these findings as not appropriate for their population, and continued with practices that seemed to work for them.

The foundation of the Royal College of General Practitioners was a landmark in the development of primary care research, emphasizing the separateness of the discipline, and the different problems posed in researching it. The work of the RCGP Birmingham Research Unit (National Morbidity Surveys), the Manchester Research Unit (Oral Contraceptive Study) and the MRC General Practice Research Framework have illustrated the usefulness of multi-practice research. Observations in single practices have made major contributions to the literature however, e.g. epidemiology of infectious hepatitis and of Bornholm's epidemic myalgia described by Pickles,[2] and the variation in general practitioners' referral rates to hospital was demonstrated first in one practice.[3] More recently, Beale[4] has reported the effects of unemployment on the health of his practice population.

The formation of university departments of general practice/primary care has been a major step towards establishing a research base for primary care. The functions of these academic units have been defined as: involvement in patient care at the highest possible standard; furtherance of the subject by research; and teaching with the twin purposes of encouraging a spirit of enquiry amongst undergraduates and of providing for the training and postgraduate development of future academic practitioners of the subject.[5] In reality, it has been usual for the academic units to be so underfunded and understaffed that there has been little opportunity to do much more than provide undergraduate teaching and a small research portfolio. Recent increases in funding have improved this situation somewhat. A national Centre for Research and Development in Primary Care has been established in Manchester with a view to developing general practice research and training researchers.

Need for primary care and interface research

General practice is the largest single branch of medicine, there being about twice as many principals in general practice as there are consultants in all

---

Box 8.1: Need for primary care and interface research

- volume of patient care undertaken in primary care
- lack of effectiveness studies in primary care populations
- shift to pro-active care
- chronic care taken over from hospital out-patients
- closure of long-stay psychiatric hospitals
- fundholding and commissioning of care
- patients' charter – increased accountability
- earlier discharge from hospital following surgery
- increased shared care and outreach clinics
- increased open-access to hospital investigations

---

the other specialities put together.[1] Almost 90% of all clinical problems are managed in general practice without referral to hospital.

Many of the interventions in primary care are based on the results of trials carried out on hospital patients, and some are based on observations from uncontrolled and unblinded case-series, carried out before the invention of the randomized controlled trial. This is not to say that the care is ineffective. It does mean that we do not have rigorous evidence that it is more effective than other interventions, or even than no intervention at all. This may have cost implications, and at worst may lead to harm being done to patients. An example of the danger of extrapolating research findings from one population to another is given in Box 8.2.

Box 8.2: Extrapolating research findings – a cautionary tale

Studies on pre-term and sick babies in special-care baby units showed that nursing them on their fronts (prone) increased the oxygenation of their blood. This, together with an unproven assumption that babies would be less likely to inhale vomit if prone, led to campaigns to encourage mothers to put **all** babies on their fronts to sleep. Studies in the community subsequently showed that sleeping prone was associated with an increased risk of cot death. Campaigns to reverse this advice, and a decrease in the number of infants sleeping prone, have been followed by a reduction in the number of cot deaths.[6]

Changing work patterns

The shift in emphasis to pro-active care has increased workload by increasing both the number of contacts for screening and the number of patients with recognized chronic problems. The majority of these patients, e.g. with hypertension, asthma, depression, are now managed in primary care[1] by an increasing number of health professionals. In addition, early discharge from hospital increases primary care workload further.

The policy of closing long-stay hospitals, particularly mental hospitals, means that primary care teams must now provide medical care for the more seriously disabled chronic sick. This implies training and resource needs, as well as increased liaison with other care providers.

Purchasers and providers

The paper *Developing NHS Purchasing and GP Fundholding – Towards a Primary Care-led NHS*[7] stresses the importance of health authorities and general practitioners working together to plan and develop health services. Fundholding, and the commissioning of care by general practitioners, puts extra responsibility on them to ensure that the care they are providing and buying is cost effective. It is increasingly important for general practitioners to know what the health needs of their population are. Methods of determining these need to be researched and evaluated.

These changes require research on the best way to provide services, as well as on the effectiveness of various interventions.

Patients' charter

There is an ever increasing demand for health care from an increasingly well-informed public. The expectation of high-quality services has been reinforced by patients' charters. The unproved interventions of previous times are no longer acceptable to patients who require to be informed of their conditions and the efficacy of treatments.

Interface

Many of these changes in primary care also involve the primary–secondary care interface. Referral of patients to hospital depends on many factors, including the resources available to deal with conditions in primary care, the current thinking on optimum management, the patient's wishes and the decision-making of the individual general practitioner. Changes in referral rates have resource implications for primary and secondary care, as does the early discharge of patients back to the community. Open-access to hospital services for the patients of general practitioners and consultant out-reach clinics in the community may make for quicker and more convenient services to patients, but may not be the most cost-effective way of using these resources.

What has primary care research to offer?

Primary care teams, centred around the registered population of general practitioners, are well placed to carry out research on populations of patients as well as on individuals. More than 90% of the total population is registered with a general practitioner, and about 80% of these see their GP each year. A drawback in inner city practices is the high rate of patient turnover. This makes it more difficult to establish a stable denominator for population studies, and to follow up individual patients. Patient tagging through the NHS central register can be used to overcome the latter problem.

General practice records contain a wealth of morbidity data, albeit in a rather unrefined state, which limits its usefulness at present. More than 80% of general practices are now computerized, potentially providing ready access to these data. Computer systems are mainly under-used, but could potentially be a major resource for research. Many GPs carry out audit in their practices, which not only gives them opportunity to learn about data collection, but can help in the introduction of protocols based on research evidence.

Recognition of the importance of observational and qualitative work by primary care practitioners in their own practices should not be lost in the pursuit of the goal of 'generalizability'. The general practitioner is ideally placed to observe the natural history of conditions, as Pickles[2] pointed out, and also the effects of treatments on individuals. This work can question accepted (but often un-evaluated) modes of practice, and inform larger studies to assess the effectiveness of particular interventions.

Problems of primary care research

Perhaps the major difficulties facing primary care researchers arise from the previous lack of a research culture throughout the discipline. Primary care is service oriented and patient centred. General practitioners run their own businesses, and must make a profit. Activities which do not bring in money tend to have a low priority. These factors affect both the undertaking of research and the implementation of research findings. Many would-be primary care researchers have probably had no training in research methods and are unable to free themselves from their service commitments for sufficient time to undertake either the training or a research project. It is difficult for researchers with no track record to obtain funding for their projects anyway and proposals which are hurriedly put together by untrained workers are almost certain to be rejected.

Box 8.3: Problems of primary care research

- lack of research culture
- heavy service commitments
- lack of research training opportunities
- difficulty obtaining funding
- difficulty maintaining recruitment to studies
- standardization of 'diagnosis'
- variation between practices
- independent contractor status of general practitioners

There is then the problem of persuading service workers to participate in the research. Even well-funded studies carried out by experienced workers have had problems in maintaining recruitment of patients. Studies on general practice may be seen to be threatening, or impractical or irrelevant if the researchers have not had sufficient advice from 'hands on' practitioners.

Many patients seen in general practice do not fit into definite disease categories. It is often more useful to think in terms of symptom complexes. It is important to define precisely the conditions needed for inclusion of patients in a study. Even so, there is an element of clinical judgement exercised by the doctor as to the eligibility of each patient, and the more doctors there are recruiting to the study, the wider will be the variation in those included. Recruitment to the study will be biased by factors such as ease of access to the primary care team (e.g. open surgeries versus appointment systems) and local cultural health beliefs about the nature of the problem and its appropriateness for medical care.

Studies of service delivery in primary care are subject to similar problems. A comparison of two systems running parallel in one practice means that other service factors are constant, but there are the problems of small numbers, lack of generalizability and 'contamination' of one group by the other e.g. patients talking between groups and wanting the other system. If the two systems are compared in different practices however, there are many confounding variables to bias the results. Many of these can be approximately matched, but practice 'philosophy' and personalities of the workers involved are not so amenable to control.

Problems in implementing research knowledge in practice

Problems with the implementation of research findings in practice are not peculiar to primary care, but some are more pertinent because of the relative isolation of many primary care practitioners and the closer relationship they may have with the patient.

The problem of deciding on the most effective interventions on the basis of research evidence applies to all health professionals. It is well recognized that this task is far beyond the scope of a single individual. The initiatives of the Cochrane Centre and the York Centre for Reviews and Dissemination should provide accurate and easily accessible information. Even so, the 'grey zones' of clinical practice[8] still greatly exceed the areas of (relative) certainty. Personal knowledge derived from experience, and clinical reasoning based on knowledge of pathophysiology, guide most medical decision making, as does patient preference. Naylor[8] points out that 'We become confident in our educated guesswork to the point where it is easy to confuse personal opinion with evidence, or personal ignorance with genuine scientific uncertainty.'

It is not easy for the practitioner to sort out the sound, evidence-based guidelines from the mass of information he or she is bombarded with each week, which includes 'evidence' from commercial companies, and guidelines from consensus statements rather than rigorous literature review.

Knowledge of research findings alone is not sufficient to change practice. The professional must believe that the research findings are relevant to his

---

Box 8.4: Problems in implementing research knowledge in practice

- knowledge not easily available/information overload
- incomplete and/or misleading reviews
- uncertainty about applicability of research findings
- unfamiliarity with new methods
- lack of contact between researchers and clinicians
- lack of resources
- organizational factors
- patient preferences

---

patients and that changing practice will increase patient benefit without increasing risk to the patient. General practitioners are still judged in law by the standard of what a 'general practitioner of ordinary skills' would have done. Fear of stepping out of line may therefore delay the adoption of a new procedure which may have some risk.

Lack of contact between researchers and clinicians can result in research not being driven by the needs of clinical practice, thus decreasing its relevance.[9] The way that delivery of care is organized may work against the implementation of research findings, as may inadequate resources.

There is great emphasis on patient-centredness in training of primary care professionals. Patients may prefer to continue with familiar treatments that they are satisfied with rather than change to something new.

Encouraging primary care research

Box 8.5 lists some of the initiatives intended to stimulate primary care research.

The document *Research for Health*[10] mentions the need for managers and clinicians to be aware of the relevance of research and development, the principles of its conduct and the potential practical gains from it, but recognizes that training opportunities need to be expanded.

Project work now features in the training of primary care professionals, and for general practitioners the written submission of practical work will form part of the end-point summative assessment. This work might be

---

Box 8.5: Initiatives intended to stimulate primary care research

- research appreciation included in training for all
- availability of research methods courses/higher degree courses
- availability of funding
- practice networks
- opportunities for release from service commitment
- research fellowships
- expansion of academic units

---

expected to foster research appreciation, but to do so it requires skilled supervision. An unsuccessful project is likely to have a negative effect. A survey of trainees and trainers in one region (undertaken by the author) revealed that 40% of trainees and 20% of trainers did not think project work was valuable, and one-fifth of trainers did not think that they could provide adequate supervision for trainees' projects. An additional problem is the short period of training for general practice which does not allow time for training in research methods. Research traineeships would be one way of encouraging trainees with an interest in research, and a few such posts are now available.

Research training opportunities for established GPs are inadequate at present, although they are increasing. Several universities now run Masters courses for primary care workers which include training in research methods. Regions offer research training fellowships, but few of them go to primary care professionals. Both these options require time away from service commitments, which can be particularly difficult for GPs. Short courses on research methods are available at a few centres, but these cannot provide the continuing support needed throughout the undertaking of a research project. This need has been met in a few regions by the establishment of networks of practices interested in research. The activities and successes of one of these are outlined in Box 8.6. The Northern Research Network owes much to the work of an RCGP Research Fellow, Dr. Pali Hungin, and was originally funded by Northern Region.

The idea of designated research practices, selected for the research abilities of the principals and their data handling facilities, has been

---

Box 8.6: The Northern Research Network (NoReN)

Aim – to enable service general practitioners and other members of the primary care team to develop their research ideas and skills and encourage them to carry out research

Activities – research training courses, research development workshops, help with applications for funding, technical help, peer support, research presentation day, higher degree support group, administrative infrastructure

Achievements – over 100 members, success in grant applications, publications, gaining of research training fellowships, good attendance at courses and seminars

---

promoted by the RCGP.[11] These would receive extra funding to free the principals from service commitment in order to carry out research and research training. Ten practices per old region was suggested as an initial target. At the time of writing (April 1995) two such practices have been appointed.

The problem of the serious underfunding of research in general practice and the community has been addressed in the Culyer report (*see* Chapter 5). The proposals in this report include the abolition of the Service Increment for Teaching and Research (SIFTR) and the creation of a single funding stream, to which primary care researchers would have increased access. Purchasers will receive increased allocations but will contribute to the research funding, so that they will have a direct interest in the research and development process. These proposals are intended to rectify the present problem of lack of co-ordination between funders, which can lead to duplication and lack of knowledge about what research is being done. This should ease the problem of 'protocol fatigue' experienced by many researchers because of the present need to make repeated applications, wasting a great deal of valuable researchers' time.

Research at the interface of primary and secondary care

Prior to the setting up of the CRDC Advisory Group to identify research and development priorities for interface research, there was no nationally co-ordinated approach. In their briefing document, the Advisory Group pointed out the need for a wide range of research methods, and for research to be undertaken by multi-disciplinary teams, including nurses, professions allied to medicine, managers, health service researchers, hospital specialists and general practitioners. The need for a consumer perspective, including the views of carers as well as patients was pointed out. Twenty-one areas of research need were outlined initially, including the areas of referral patterns, information transfer, access to diagnostic facilities, effects of increasing day-case surgery and shorter hospital admissions, shared-care, prescribing, impact of purchasing arrangements, and the changing skills and training needs at the interface.

Implementing research findings in primary care

The strategies for implementing research knowledge in practice are largely the same in primary care as in other branches of medicine, and may be divided into patient-centred, educational, administrative and economic.[9]

Informing patients about the effectiveness of interventions through the media or specific campaigns can be a powerful way of influencing the practitioner. On the other hand, patients may reject new ideas in favour of familiar interventions that they believe in.

General practitioners are expected to spend five days each year on accredited continuing education, and a part of their income depends on their providing evidence that they have done so. There is very little published work to show that this education makes any difference to patient outcomes. It has been suggested that discussion of practice guidelines, and audit of how they are implemented, should be more closely linked to continuing medical education.[9]

Computer systems that incorporate guidelines provide accessible information, and there is evidence that patient specific reminders lead to higher use of guidelines.

The application of marketing principles has been suggested for health care development.[12] 'Top down' approaches of implementing guidelines are product-oriented rather than consumer-oriented. The marketing approach, by focusing on the needs of the 'consumer' (clinician) and developing and promoting a knowledge 'product' that meets those needs, may be more effective. This might increase the contact between researcher and clinician and as a result lead to research being more relevant to the needs of the NHS.

Economic incentives have already been used in primary care in the form of target payments for high levels of immunization and uptake of cervical cytology. There is also payment for the chronic care of diabetes and asthma according to approved protocols, and for health promotion activities. Future economic pressure to implement effective care and discontinue ineffective interventions may be applied by purchasers of care.

Guidelines for management of conditions should be applied only to those patients in whom a relatively certain diagnosis can be made. Whilst the implementation of proven best practice is of great importance, it must be remembered that this evidence is not available for many areas of practice[8] and probably more than half of the patients seen in primary care do not fit into neat diagnostic categories.

Summary

The recognition of the importance of primary care in the NHS, and the changing interface between primary and secondary care, have drawn attention to the relative lack of high quality research in these areas. The reasons for this include lack of training, time and funding for would-be primary care researchers. Expansion of university departments of primary care, increased opportunities for primary care professionals to obtain higher degrees, research fellowships, research practices, and proposed changes in funding are among the initiatives to promote research in primary care. Audit, informed by evidence-based guidelines, may be useful in the implementation of research findings. Purchasing may also be used to encourage effective practice. For these initiatives to be successful, research appreciation must be included in the training of all primary care professionals, not as an optional extra but as an underlying concept throughout training.

References

1 Pereira Gray D (1991) Research in general practice: law of inverse opportunity. *British Medical Journal*, **302**:1380–2.
2 Pickles W (1939) *Epidemiology in Country Practice*. RCGP, London.
3 Morrell DC, Gage HG and Robinson N. (1971) Referral to hospital by general practitioners. *Journal of the Royal College of General Practitioners*, **21**:77–85.

4 Beale N, Nethercott S (1987) The health of industrial employees four years after compulsory redundancy. *Journal of the Royal College of General Practitioners,* **37**:390–4.

5 Morrell DC (1979) Now and then. William Pickles lecture. *Journal of the Royal College of General Practitioners,* **29**:457–65.

6 Department of Health (1993) *Report of the Chief Medical Officer's Expert Group on The Sleeping Position of Infants and Cot Death.* HMSO, London.

7 NHS Executive (1994) *Developing NHS Purchasing and GP Fundholding– Towards a Primary Care-led NHS.* Department of Health, London.

8 Naylor DC (1995) Grey zones of clinical practice: some limits to evidence-based medicine. *The Lancet,* **345**:840–2.

9 Haines A and Jones R (1994) Implementing findings of research. *British Medical Journal,* **308**:1488–92.

10 Peckham M (1993) *Research for Health.* Department of Health, London.

11 The Conference of Academic Organizations in General Practice (1994) *Research and General Practice.* RCGP, London.

12 Dickinson E (1995) Using marketing principles for healthcare development. *Quality in Health Care,* **4**:40–4.

9

Managing research and development

ANTONY J FRANKS

Introduction

Research within the NHS has historically reflected the interests of the research community with any benefit, both potential and realized, to the NHS (in terms of its main function of caring for patients) being haphazard.

Central to the NHS research and development strategy is the need to actively manage the processes whereby research needs are identified, research aspirations harnessed and research findings acted on so that patients derive maximum benefit from them. This is the purpose of research management. It aims to convert ideas, enthusiasm, skills and experience from the research community into knowledge relevant to the practice and needs of the NHS.

The chain of events linking the initiation of research and the eventual translation of research findings into practice is complex; whilst, traditionally, research initiation, the decision to fund and the implementation of results have been separate (intellectually and temporally), successful project management should encompass all three.

Reactive or commissioned research?

Researcher-led versus strategy-led

Research can be broadly separated into that which is driven by the interests of the researcher for which funding is then sought (reactive or responsive funding) and that which is driven by the wish of the funder to address specific topics or questions relevant to their needs (commissioned research). These two are not mutually exclusive but represent complementary approaches; they differ not so much in the type of project management but in its timing. The following consideration of project management will largely focus on commissioned research but, as will become apparent, the principles will be applicable to reactive research.

Clarifying the objective

In order to commission research a funding body must have a strategic view of its research needs and also be able to translate this strategic view into explicit priority areas, topics or research questions. For example 'cancer of the lung' might be a priority area by virtue of its frequency and morbidity, 'effective therapy for small cell carcinoma of the lung' might be a defined topic, and 'what is the value of current measures of likelihood of benefit from intensive chemotherapy for small-cell lung cancer?' would be a specific research question.

Priority setting

The process of priority setting is a complex one involving iterative consideration of possibilities in the light of a number of explicit parameters. These will include:

- the value to the NHS of the answer to the question
- the potential impact on the public health of the research result
- the practicability of research in the area
- existing research expertise
- the relationship of the topic to existing policy priorities.

Priority setting has usually involved panels of individuals whose backgrounds and expertise reflect these parameters; another strategy for identifying potential priority areas is the commissioning of reviews of a topic where research needs may exist. This stage should include consideration of existing research which may yield results relevant to the priority, research under discussion and completed research whose results have yet to be published or converted into practice.

Where the research priority, and the research questions, stem from an identified need to achieve change the early involvement of the agents for change and those from whom change will be sought will increase the likelihood of a commitment to act on the findings (see the case history below). There is however a price to be paid and that is that the process will inevitably take longer.

Commissioning research

Once priorities are established researchers must be sought to conduct the work. In principle this will be a process whereby there is a conjunction between a desired research outcome and a local capacity to conduct the necessary research.

In practice this can be achieved by a variety of mechanisms which can be visualized as a spectrum. At one extreme is a general invitation to the research community to apply for funds. At the other end a specific researcher, or research group, could be asked to conduct a specified piece of work.

Graded steps within this spectrum could be conceptualized as:

- a generalized invitation to engage in competitive submission within a specified priority area

- a generalized invitation to engage in competitive submission for specific projects within a specified priority area

- a generalized invitation to submit for specific projects within a specified priority area with the opportunity to revise the proposal after initial consideration

- a specific invitation to a researcher, or group, to submit for specific projects within a specified priority area with the opportunity to revise the proposal after initial consideration

- a specific invitation to a researcher, or group, to design and deliver a specific research project.

In all these situations quality criteria would apply but the degree to which the process is competitive and the point at which a funding decision is made would differ.

Commissioning research has advantages in that it is more likely to result in research relevant to the funders' needs. On the other hand it requires clearer agendas for research and good knowledge of available research skills and facilities. The commissioning body's intentions must be clear to intending applicants as an initial stage in ensuring that the research proposals received are relevant to their needs.

Commissioning research – a case history

October 1993

A clinical research subgroup of the regional R&D office identified the need to examine the implementation of existing and increasing new knowledge of the treatment of acute myocardial infarction based on the results of recent large-scale clinical trials. An initial approach was made to the chairman of the regional cardiology group.

November 1993

The chairman in turn wrote to all regional cardiologists.

January 1994

A generally favourable response was elicited.

February 1994

The research manager wrote suggesting that the proposal be developed with the help of an epidemiologist with expertise in this field.

March 1994

A small steering group made up of representatives of the regional cardiology group, an academic cardiologist and an epidemiologist was set up. The first draft of their proposal was produced for discussion with the research manager. The proposal, whilst broadly in line with the intent of the funding body had concentrated on a study of the means of ascertaining the event (acute myocardial infarction) based on coronary care units, without incorporating the issue of determining current practice.

April 1994

The project was referred back for modification, and support from regional cardiologists for the modified project was secured. This was an essential step since the project would involve access to data in all Coronary Care Units in the region and examination of treatment. The proposal differed from audit in that it set out:

● to determine the most efficient means of identifying patients in whom treatment could be studied

- to identify local protocols for treatment and

- to define the degree to which these protocols determined practice.

May 1994

The first full draft of the costed proposal was submitted and considered by the R&D group. Further review of statistical aspects of the study followed with development of a full protocol incorporating comparative data acquisition methods.

May – November 1994

Two further development meetings were held between the research manager, the epidemiologist and the cardiologist who were developing the proposal, before the final proposal was submitted.

December 1994

The final proposal was approved for funding after external peer review.

March 1995

There was some modification in the light of the reviewer's advice and project workers were appointed for a two year period.

Key points

Commissioning research can be time consuming if the success of that research depends (as here) on the support of a large regional group of clinicians. On the other hand the conduct of the research is likely to have been greatly facilitated by their early involvement and later problems regarding data access are less likely (see problems below); this project straddles R&D examining practice and means of determining it, and will give insights into ways of facilitating implementation.

Project management

This is a valuable function which has greatly enhanced the quality and standing of the R&D process in many NHS regions in England and Wales. Despite a belief that the involvement of research managers in the research process would be viewed negatively by the research community, who might have seen this as a threat to their scientific independence and credibility, informal feed-back from funded researchers has been generally positive.

The importance attached to project management is such that it is included in the full definition of NHS R&D (see Chapter 1, Box 1.4). In its fullest form project management ensures that a continuity exists between the initial proposal, the project structure and its development and the aims of the body allocating funding. There are potential and realized savings by this process of project modification. In offering guidance to applicants during negotiations over their project, research management should contribute directly to the educational role of regional R&D activity in that it impinges on project design and the actual practice of research.

The process of active research management is too recently introduced to see any effects in terms of outcome but in conjunction with a more critical selection process geared to the needs of the NHS the expectation that a higher proportion of research projects will yield results of value to the NHS is a reasonable one; the process compares favourably with the old locally-organized research scheme (LORS) where in one year (1992) in one representative region only one half of projects actually submitted definitive final reports. The relevance of these to the NHS was not assessed although it has been estimated that only about 30% of such projects would have been relevant to the Health of the Nation.

The research manager is a bridge between commissioner and researcher. He/she is responsible for ensuring that the commissioner's intentions in funding the project are achieved; the research manager should be providing such support and advice as is necessary to drive the research to a successful conclusion while, at the same time, ensuring the interests of the funder are safeguarded. This will involve initial confirmation of the quality of the intended research (is it capable of answering the questions being posed?) and the practicability of the proposal (is it adequately resourced in terms of skills and finances?). This stage is essential whether the decision is on a commissioned project or a reactive one.

Project selection

The process of decision-making on research proposals is one for which there are no clear rules or methods of proven validity (in terms of the value of the end result). While methods differ they will have in common the following:

- the use of a group rather than an individual

- the expectation that those involved in the process will bring relevant skills to bear on the decision

- that where relevant skills or knowledge are not available these will be sought from outside the group (for instance by the use of external referees).

Key parameters in the decision-making process should include:

- the validity of the scientific basis for the proposal (*a sine qua non*)

- the potential value to the NHS of the product from the proposed research.

Supplementary issues will include a judgement on the likelihood that the research will be successful in achieving its objectives (this is not the same as proving a hypothesis); account should be taken of the experience and track record of the applicants. Where the project is deemed to be of importance, but the researchers less experienced, the degree of support through project management will need to be greater.

The process has to be administered (in terms of ensuring that the relevant papers get to the relevant people in an agreed time scale) but must also be managed so that the criteria on which decisions will be made are explicit and can be operationalized in a realistic way to allow a decision to be reached. Decisions will range from one not to fund through to one to fund the proposal as presented. In practice the latter will be rare since there will usually be gaps between the researchers' proposal and the funder's intentions. These may be based on the science or the focus and both can be subject to modification and review before a project is finally funded or rejected. This is a time-consuming process for both parties and a two-stage process has much to commend it.

In a two-stage process a short initial proposal is submitted which, in essence, presents a project outline in sufficient detail to allow funders to determine whether the research is potentially capable of meeting their needs. This approach reduces the time needed to produce and to consider the proposal. Applicants successful at the end of the first stage are asked to submit a far more detailed proposal, usually within a stated time scale, which will take account of specific issues raised by the funder. These may include concerns about statistical power, the wish to see other aspects included or certain aspects excluded, and the possibility of collaboration with others in the same field (who may have submitted complementary but competing bids).

The nature and degree of input from the funder will vary with the level of resources committed to this activity and the nature of the changes sought by the funder from the researchers. Thus advice from specialists on design and analysis issues or health economics may be made available. Some regions have established research support units where specialists provide advice to intending applicants.

At the second stage discussion can be focused on the questions of practicability and the validity of the scientific basis for the proposal since the initial question of whether the project is relevant to the funder's needs has already been settled. In practice there will be debate about the relative merits of projects where resources are limited but this approach, whilst it means that decisions will take longer, is more likely to result in projects relevant to the NHS; incorporating the funder's concerns is also easier at this stage than later (when things are far less flexible). The time of all concerned is used to far greater effect, in terms of achieving a research strategy, than the more traditional approach of dividing a defined cake according to the relative merits of those proposals which. have been received by a given deadline.

Agreement to fund is an important stage but may still leave items for clarification before the final commitment, in terms of a contract, between researcher, or more usually their institution, and funder is signed. This will specify the level and period of funding, and will also detail the agreement on who owns any intellectual property; the latter would generally belong to the NHS unless there is an element of joint funding or there has been prior agreement to alternative arrangements.

Pilot studies

The commonest problems encountered in project monitoring (see below) relate to recruitment of sufficient patients in a clinical study or access to data for a health services research study. In both these cases the agreement to fund could build in the requirement of a pilot phase with lower funding levels; during this period the practicability of the proposal and solutions to the almost inevitable problems can be clearly identified. This is, in practice, rarely done and many initial study periods are, in effect, unplanned pilot phases which result in inevitable alterations to plans and timing. They are usually left out of research proposals because their inclusion would mean that the period of research, or its costs, fall outside limits set by the funder. It is uncertain whether such limits have any value other than contributing to the gamble that the funder may get the research done for a lower cost against the likelihood that to get the work done (with project management) will require the implementation of solutions which will involve extra expenditure of time or money or both.

Financial arrangements

There is a legitimate concern that funds committed to NHS R&D should be well controlled, used for the purpose for which they have been allocated, and be accountable. To ensure this it is necessary to establish effective systems for financial control at project level which achieve these ends without being unnecessarily bureaucratic or burdensome.

The NHS (for these purposes the R&D section of a Regional office of the Management Executive) will make the commitment to fund a piece of work. The researcher will identify a financial administrator in their organization who will be responsible, on a day-to-day basis for the payment of bills associated with the project. That financial administrator will then arrange to recharge (usually in arrears on a quarterly basis) the Regional office for the sums incurred in the preceding period. The fact that the NHS accounts on a financial year basis means that track should be kept of project spending to prevent a build-up of unspent commitment in any one year. Depending on the local arrangements this may be part of the arrangements for project management or may be handled by separate financial mechanisms.

Although agreement to fund is for a stated period and for a stated sum it is essential that there is sufficient flexibility to allow for response to changed circumstances. If the project involves the employment of staff the contract will recognize that nationally-agreed salary increases will be paid by effectively increasing the sum committed. There is no universal practice over the payment of overheads.

Overheads

The costs of any research project are made up of:

1   Costs which are easily, solely and directly attributable to the project such as salary of research workers, laboratory and office consumables, travelling expenses, specific equipment etc.

2   Costs which are relatively easily attributable to the project but which may pay for goods or services which are occasionally used for other

purposes such as secretarial time, equipment necessary for the project but with wider application, telephone costs etc.

3   Costs which are incurred by the host organization as a consequence of the presence of the project but which would, to a greater or lesser extent, be incurred anyway such as library facilities, heating, lighting, accommodation, central computing facilities etc.

In establishing the costs of any project those in 1 are easily quantifiable, those in 2 are relatively easily quantifiable, if subject to agreement on apportionment of cost to be borne by the funding body; those in 3 are usually referred to, and sought as, overheads. There are two perspectives on overheads:

- those of the funding agency which, among other things, seeks value in terms of research results in return for its investment

- those of the host organization which seeks to further its research ability and reputation (which have implications for future allocation of central funding) whilst at the same time recovering from whatever available source the costs of maintaining these and its broader range of activities.

The problem is one which combines principle (who should pay for what benefit?) and a decision about the equitable apportionment of financial burden. As financial pressures on both funding and recipient organizations have increased so the custom and practice of routine payment of overheads has begun to break down. Some funding agencies pay no overheads and, where overheads are paid, there is a wide range of percentages sought by different institutions. These issues are brought into a sharper focus with the increasing move from reactive to commissioned research. It can be argued that where the funder approaches an organization, unit or project team in order to achieve a research aim the benefit might lie more with the funder than the recipient; as such the obligation to meet overheads in a situation more akin to a contractual arrangement is higher. Counter to that view is the fact that, in agreeing to undertake research, a recipient organization will do so knowing that its reputation and other functions (such as teaching) will be enhanced and that this will lead to wider but less immediately quantifiable benefits.

Monitoring progress

Once agreement to fund is reached and the contract signed the project can begin. There may still be activity prior to the period of funding such as the recruitment of staff and final amendments to protocols. There is no general agreement on the frequency with which projects should be monitored for progress nor which is the most effective way of monitoring. It should be said that whilst project monitoring is an important part of project management the holding of regular meetings with project staff is often the only way of ensuring that all members of the research team have an opportunity to concentrate on the project in a strategic sense; in multiworker projects only one or two members of the team may be aware of what the others are doing and many research groups have commented on the benefit derived from having to meet for project management purposes.

The purpose behind project management is to ensure the successful completion of NHS funded research. It is necessary to remember that success should be judged in terms of the funder's objectives, not solely those of the researcher. It follows therefore that the funder's objectives, if explicit and clear, will determine the direction of project management; to focus exclusively on the process may not ensure that the goals inherent in the decision to fund are achieved.

It is a fallacy that the decision to fund a research proposal results in a well-designed project capable of answering the questions contained within it. In the absence of preliminary pilot or feasibility studies assumptions inherent in the original proposal may prove to be unfounded or, more usually, over-optimistic. As a result simple process measures of achievement may be taken to indicate failure when in fact they indicate the need for revision of the project structure to achieve the desired end. If that end is clearly stated and understood by the project manager it is easier to place any measure of achievement in perspective.

Most common problems arise in the first three months and it is usually necessary to meet at least once with the project team soon after agreement to fund is reached in order to define the means whereby project management will be conducted. The simplest way is by reference to agreed milestones (*see* Box 9.1).

Box 9.1: SMART milestones

- Simple
- Measurable
- Achievable
- Realistic
- Timed

These can then serve as points of reference by which progress can be assessed. The means of project monitoring will be determined by available skills and resources but should be capable of identifying problems in progress or responding to such problems identified by the researchers. This may be achieved by use of a suitably qualified/experienced research manager or by the use of regular written reports whose structure allows progress to be followed and problems identified.

Problems

Reference has already been made to difficulties with recruitment of patients in numbers sufficient to meet the sample size necessary if the project is to have sufficient statistical power (i.e. be able to answer the questions it is asking). Reasons for this are many but they frequently reflect over-optimistic estimates about the frequency of the condition under study or of the preparedness of colleagues to undertake the extra work necessary to recruit patients. Possible solutions will depend on the circumstances but include:

- extending the catchment area for patient recruitment
- extending the period of the study to allow sufficient time for sample size to be collected; this can be coupled with a reduced funding level until appropriate recruitment levels have been reached. In effect this constitutes a pilot phase which could, perhaps, have been required initially
- employment of staff dedicated to the collection of cases
- accepting a reduced study power
- cessation of project funding.

The solution chosen will depend on circumstance but will usually involve extra expenditure. This is easier to justify if the project has already passed through a selection process which has explicitly identified the subject as one which is of value to the NHS; project reviews will need to be frequent enough to measure the impact of the solution as soon as possible in order that a decision can be made whether further action is necessary. In practice this requires a quarterly review of progress, although once a project has passed its first year things are usually sufficiently stable to allow a less frequent review cycle. Although review meetings may be informal it is valuable to impose some form of structure and for formal annual review this is essential since it may constitute the only point at which members of the funding body are brought up to date with progress of individual projects. A suggested project review structure is in Box 9.2.

Box 9.2: Annual project review – suggested headings for review form

- Research questions
- Project abstract
- Milestones of achievement (from original grant application) – these should indicate expected achievements at specified times into the project
- Progress report – indicate specifically whether milestones have been achieved and, if not, give reasons and action taken in response (use additional sheets as necessary)
- Planned activity in next 12 months

Project completion

Traditionally this has involved the production of a report for the funding body and papers for publication in peer-reviewed journals. In a policy environment where the purpose of research is to inform the practice and delivery of health care other steps are needed. These will usually relate to the needs of those commissioning health care. The results of the research project may be clear and self-explanatory – a technique is effective or ineffective and should or should not be purchased on grounds of efficacy. The nature of the choice which will have to be made will have been apparent from an early stage; it is preferable therefore that the managerial, as well as clinical, significance of the research is identified while it is in progress so that the necessary steps can be taken as soon as the final analyses and conclusions have been reached. In this way the research is part of the developing policy stream while it is being carried out rather than remaining external to it until its completion. This illustrates the view that research should be embedded in development, not the sole drive to development.

Rarely is the matter as clear as this; the topic to which the research contributes may be a complex one and the significance of the results may not be self-evident; in these circumstances some form of review, probably independently commissioned, will be necessary to place the research findings in context. It is almost always the case that the final analyses, and certainly the report, are delayed beyond the period of funding. If the project has been successfully managed it is possible to distinguish those projects whose results have a need for further action from those which do not, and act accordingly. What is often less obvious is who should be informed about the results of research. An output aimed at the readers of peer-reviewed journals will satisfy the legitimate career and scientific aspirations of the researchers but often as much value can be obtained by asking the researchers 'Given your area of expertise what do these results mean and who do you think should know about them?'

Conclusion

Research funded by the NHS should be actively managed to ensure that projects are of high quality in terms of structure, process and outcome. The level of management should be commensurate with the scale and complexity of the project, the experience of the researchers, the potential importance of the result and available resources.

10

Implementing the results of research and development in clinical and managerial practice

STEPHEN HARRISON

Introduction

Implementing research and development (R&D) findings seems to be a rational thing to do: otherwise, why bother to produce the findings? Yet it is now a commonplace observation that, in the field of health care R&D at least, such implementation is by no means the norm. This has been neatly summed up by two North American observers:

> In an ideal world, there would be no gap between what is known from sound research about the means to promote health and the means actually employed by health care practitioners in administering care to their patients. In fact, however, there is a distressing distance between care knowledge in general and the practices of individual clinicians for most validated health care procedures.[1]

Whilst substantial resources are now being invested (on both sides of the Atlantic) in institutions whose function is to encourage such implementation (*see* Chapter 4) their effectiveness is as yet far from clear. Indeed, the 'implementation problem' is a complex one which is unlikely to be solved in any simplistic sense, though that is not to say that some improvement cannot be secured. Implementation problems are, of course, ubiquitous across all policy sectors and there exists a general literature upon which this chapter draws in order to illuminate the issues and to indicate some general lessons.

This chapter is divided into four remaining sections. Each of the first three draws upon a different model of policy implementation (respectively, 'top-down', 'bottom-up' and 'strategic') adapted from the work of Majone and Wildavsky.[2] The final section draws some conclusions and sets out their implications for policy on implementing R&D findings.

The top-down model: implementation as control

Top-down models of policy implementation work from the premise that there exists an appropriate policy, determined in the upper reaches of the organization's hierarchy, and that the key task thereafter is to have the policy implemented as thoroughly as possible. Implementation is therefore a control issue and this model can be approached by setting out the conditions that would have to be met if thorough or 'perfect' implementation were to occur.[3] In the present case, there seem to be seven such conditions, which are set out in Box 10.1.

Box 10.1: A top-down model of implementation of R&D findings in health care

The following seven conditions would *all* have to be met for 'perfect implementation' of evidence-based standards of professional practice in any specific area of health care:

1 the existence of normative statements, based upon relevant research, about health care professional practice

2 the ability of such statements to be interpreted as more-or-less unequivocal indications of both (a) a class of patient, and (b) a 'treatment' for such patients

3 the dissemination of these statements to all professionals likely to encounter the relevant class of patient

4 adequate (material and non-material) resources to professionals to perform the appropriate treatments or services

5 adequate (intrinsic and/or extrinsic) incentives for most relevant professionals to comply with the norms

6 the absence of substantial (material or non-material) organizational disincentives to comply with the norms

7 adequate co-ordination of a chain or team of actors which is not so large as to render the total probability of their compliance unacceptably small.

Source: S. Harrison (1994). Knowledge into practice: what's the problem? *Journal of Management in Medicine,* **8**:(2).

Setting out the conditions in this way makes it brutally clear how unlikely it is that anything approaching such thorough implementation will ever occur. Something will be said about each of these in turn.

Normative statements

Those involved in specifying appropriate technologies naturally wish their specifications to be as authoritative as possible. Broadly, there are two approaches to this. One is the provision of authoritative statements by experts, based on reviews of research evidence; the ideal standards for such guidelines are summarized by Grimshaw and Russell.[4] The alternative is the use of consensus conferences, or similar procedures aimed at securing agreement amongst interested parties. Grimshaw and Russell have questioned the authority of guidelines drawn up by experts, whilst the sheer range of treatment types and patient subgroups to be found in a modern health service, together with the rate of technological development makes it unlikely that a comprehensive range of guidelines could ever be developed.

Unequivocality

A number of commentators have expressed the concern that supposed guidelines are not necessarily unequivocal. Thus, a recent *Lancet* editorial[5] alleged that consensus is frequently achieved by compromise, rather than unanimity, and the use of vague or general language with which it is difficult to disagree. Similarly, a group of researchers commented that, in the context of the United States, 'We found that it was often difficult to determine which practices were being recommended, and to which patient populations they applied.'[6]

It is not difficult to imagine that the same lack of specificity characterizes more local attempts to set standards; researchers have noted the tendency for audit criteria to be implicit rather than explicit.[7] At the same time, locally set standards are likely to have greater effect than nationally set ones, yet are less likely to be based on the greatest expertise.[8,9]

Dissemination

Dissemination strategies for guidelines about appropriate technology have, by contrast, been the topic of substantial research.[1,8,10,11,12] The conclusions of these reviews are highly consonant with each other.

Most effective in changing behaviour are likely to be patient-specific reminders aimed at the specific clinician, perhaps in the form of an on-line computer prompt at the point of consultation. Likely to be somewhat less effective in these terms is patient-specific feedback (perhaps through audit, continuing medical education, or 'preceptorship' by an educationally-influential person) or a 'product champion' removed in time from the consultation. The less clinician-specific and patient-specific the intervention, the less likely it is to be effective in changing behaviour; general mailings and academic or professional journal publications fall into this category, and are most likely to impact upon those clinicians already nearest to the standard of appropriateness.

Adequate resources

The relationship between the efficacy of health care interventions (that is, their results in ideal conditions) and their effectiveness when applied to the average patient by the average practitioner in average circumstances, is currently a UK national research priority, and it may be expected that such work will uncover skill and physical resource deficits that inhibit appropriate changes in professional behaviour.

However one area in which more general sociological research into the activities of professions highlights is that of time as a resource. Thus researchers such as Lipsky[13] and his colleagues have seen the work of occupations such as medicine, nursing, social work and police work as characterized by an infinity of possible workload. As a result, it is argued, 'cutting corners' is an endemic feature of professionalism, exemplified by over-hasty diagnosis or 'labelling' of the client; this categorization then functions as a guide to action or therapy.[14] Melia's study of nursing graphically illustrated how constant pressure to get the work done leads to an emphasis upon doing physical work rather than thinking about the work.[15]

Moreover, there is a view, though it is not clear how widespread, that professional time in the NHS is increasingly under pressure from management-related changes in the NHS; a recent study of obstacles to the medical audit process noted that:

Lack of time was exacerbated by other concurrent health service reforms that had led to an increase in demands on consultants' time. Activities such as resource management and collecting clinical information all imposed their own load. Thus, although the introduction of audit officers and assistants was generally appreciated, it was felt that there was still insufficient time for analysing results and preparing for meetings. As a result, seeing more patients or spending more time teaching juniors were viewed by some consultants as possibly more effective uses of their time.[16]

Incentives

It is clear that one cannot simply assume the motivation to implement R&D findings. Practitioners may fear for the initiative and autonomy that characterizes their profession:

> There was a common, recurring perception that audit sought to turn medical practice from an individualized, subtle art into an unthinking, routine activity based largely on guidelines and rules. Many doctors believed that such dependency upon guidelines would have adverse effects for doctors, destroying the initiative of juniors who would no longer think through the logistics of treatment but pick up a form and tick the appropriate box.[16]

Professionals may therefore lack the intrinsic motivation to change behaviour. But they may need extrinsic motivation too. The most pervasive form of extrinsic motivation is money and policymakers who seek to influence medical behaviour have rarely shrunk from its use; curiously, though, the same behavioural assumptions are less often made about other professionals. Success in the use of direct financial incentives for doctors has been reported in a number of studies[17] and the response of British GPs to target payments for vaccination and immunization and cervical cytology is widely held as a further demonstration. At the same time, however, little is known about the shape of incentive curves applicable to doctors, making the assumption that an array of compliance behaviours can be made dependent upon direct financial incentives a dangerous one; it is possible, for instance, that they may have a target income, with the result that increased financial incentives would cause reduced compliance efforts.[18]

There seems to be a growing assumption in Britain that indirect financial incentives, i.e. to the institution, rather than the professional, will have the same effect; this underpins aspirations that the purchaser/ provider split in the NHS will be able to function as the catalyst for the diffusion of appropriate technology. There is, however, little hard evidence of this, though some researchers have noted the use by hospital managers of the threat of 'loss of business' to influence clinical behaviour.[19]

There is little evidence about intrinsic incentives, though some researchers have argued that widespread adverse media publicity may be a factor in reducing the incidence of an inappropriate technology.[6]

Disincentives

Whatever the incentives for appropriate technology, there is always the possibility that they may be wholly or partly outweighed by disincentives. There is a good deal of general organizational research which suggests that formal managerial messages about what constitutes desirable behaviour may be countermanded by covert messages which sanction quite different behaviour.[20] Though there is little significant NHS research on this topic, it is easy to translate the above general thesis into a scenario in which a hospital's management is more concerned with throughput, or the successful marketing of a new patient service, than with the appropriateness of the technology employed. Thus, senior members of the organization might be satisfied with the *appearance* of professional compliance.

> Finally, there is the danger of doctors appearing to change their clinical practice to produce better audit results while in reality continuing to practice in the same way. In one of the hospitals, a house officer admitted that juniors had decided to modify their entries in the case notes in order to influence the audit results and maintain the appearance of reaching their targets.[16]

Indeed, in some cases, employees might actually be penalized for behaving appropriately; in nursing for instance it has been shown that students who attempt to follow the tenets of their training by spending time communicating with patients, may actually be punished.[15]

Co-ordination

Not all health care is focused upon the activities of a single clinician in relation to a single patient, yet a good deal of the literature about the effectiveness of guidelines on appropriate technology implicitly assumes such a model. The problem is taken as being to change the consultant's or the GP's behaviour in respect of investigation, surgery, prescribing or referral. Indeed, given the intellectual origin of much guidelines work in the literature of medical practice variations, this is hardly surprising. In practice, of course, it may be an important element in R&D implementation that whole teams of health professionals behave in a particular way. Obvious examples of this are hospital nursing, where the twenty-four hour necessity for patient care multiples the scope for errors and omissions, and community care, which relies on a whole network of different professionals, perhaps employed by several agencies. The number of players whose co-operation is needed defines, for implementation purposes, the complexity of the technology.[21] Suppose that a particular technology requires the co-operation of a team or chain of ten persons to implement it, and suppose that the (independent) probability of each person acting appropriately is (a relatively high) 0.95. The overall probability of perfect implementation is thus 0.95 to the power of ten, or little better than evens. However, professionals are not necessarily the independent players assumed by the probability calculus set out above; indeed, a good deal of the non-health specific literature on technology diffusion stresses the importance of the social networks in promoting innovation.[22] Thus, it seems likely that peer pressure (in one direction or the other) will be an important variable in the implementation of R&D findings.

The bottom-up model: implementation as interaction

Many of the observations made in connection with the preceding 'top-down' model point towards what in some senses constitutes a more realistic approach. Thus, for instance, Lipsky's[13] characterization of the professional work can easily be seen as a description of the process by which the NHS's services are shaped: as the aggregate of individuals' clinical behaviours.[23] This is also consonant with the widely observed, but largely unexplained, phenomenon of medical practice variations.[24] In the face of such observations, it is tempting to adopt a 'bottom-up' model of implementation.

Such a model minimizes the importance of plans or goals (in this case, the aspiration of disseminating professional practice based on R&D findings), which simply become a starting point for either overt bargaining or covert adjustment[25] amongst the various actors in the policy arena. In such a situation of pluralism it makes sense to speak of policy only with hindsight[26] and the distinction between policy and implementation approaches dissolution; in addition, the significance of organizational hierarchy is dramatically reduced. One effect of such an approach may well be to minimize conflict.[27]

The limitations are, however, potentially serious. First, the most influential actors in the policy arena, who are not necessarily those for whose benefit the policy exists, are likely to benefit most; in the present context, failure to implement (sound) R&D findings will be at the aggregate expense of patients. Moreover, constant policy compromises can be the proverbial 'worst of all worlds', incurring costs without benefits. For policymakers with aspirations to change some aspect of the world for (as they perceive it) the better, bottom-up approaches to implementation represent a counsel of despair. In a health service research context, the bottom-up model is tantamount to medical syndicalism.[2]

A strategic approach: policy as disposition, implementation as evolution

Any useful model of implementation must both recognize the very serious limitations of the top-down model and yet still avoid the nihilism of the bottom-up model; it must therefore incorporate insights derived from both models whilst providing for some means of changing the world at least in the general direction intended. One might summarize many of the limitations of the top-down control model as its lack of attention to people; it adopts too great a level of abstraction from the real, and messy, world.[28] People are difficult to control directly, both because they have minds and interests of their own, and because neither they nor their would-be controllers are perfectly equipped with foresight about the consequences of their actions.

> Objectives are characteristically multiple (because we want many things, not just one), conflicting (because we want different things) and vague (because that is how we can agree to proceed without having to agree also on exactly what to do).[2]

> We can discover [problems] and incorporate them into our plans only as the implementation process unfolds.[2]

Thus, there will be substantial 'bottom-up' elements: implementation will shape policy. At the same time, however, policy *can* shape implementation and outcomes;[29] it is, after all, policy that largely determines what resources are available to whom, and the rules within which such resources can legitimately be expended. Policy is thus a disposition, not a master plan; implementation is thus a process of evolution or learning.[2]

Towards some conclusions

In the specific context of the implementation of R&D findings in health care, all this implies the need to create an organizational culture in which learning, both by clinicians and policymakers, is facilitated. This would be a different model of learning from that implied by the top-down model (learning consists of obeying guidelines) or the bottom-up model (learning is random). Such a model might draw on recent evidence[30] that suggests that clinical doctors do not think about the effectiveness of interventions in the same way as do epidemiologists and health service researchers, that is, in terms of 'certainty about probability'. Rather, such clinicians are more influenced by their own past experiences with their own patients and by the experiences of their close colleagues or mentors. (This can be seen as a perspective on the difference between efficacy and effectiveness.)

This evolutionary approach to the implementation of R&D findings would concentrate upon the creation of a provider organizational culture in which reflective clinical practice is facilitated. The centrepiece of such a culture would be a vibrant audit process in which clinicians were able to monitor and question their own practice and their own results. Such processes would inevitably be informed by R&D findings (either by their incorporation into audit standards, or as a comparator with local outcomes), but would not be dominated by the writing of guidelines or protocols into contracts.[31,32] Of course, the insights of the top-down model need to be retained; in particular the need for sufficient time and resources for audit, and the need to avoid disincentives to participate.

A great deal of academic attention has been devoted to the concept of 'organizational culture' during the last decade[32,34] and some large claims have been made about how to manipulate such cultures.[35] Unfortunately, knowledge about how to change cultures is by no means secure, *a priori*, therefore mechanisms need to be devised and tested (R&D findings should be applied to policymaking as well as to professional practice)[36] which allow policymakers (purchasers, in the present-day structure of the NHS) to satisfy themselves that the culture of health care provider organizations approximates to that outlined above.

It is not the purpose of this chapter to specify such mechanisms in detail, but it follows from the general thrust of the analysis employed so far that their implementation should itself serve as an opportunity for organizational learning. Thus choice from various approaches might be encouraged, and the different approaches subsequently evaluated. Amongst such approaches might be the following.

Accreditation approaches

If accreditation is seen as a viable option for the quasi-regulation of health care providers, it could include a sort of 'cultural audit' aimed at discovering the degree of reflectiveness incorporated in clinical behaviour.

The Health Advisory Service

The HAS has several decades of experience of assessing provider institutions on the basis of partly 'soft' standards, and is presumably capable of developing its remit further in the direction of R&D implementation.

A Health Development Agency

The distinguishing feature of a development agency is that it has resources (albeit at a modest level) available to serve as a positive incentive for behaviour changes in the desired direction.

These suggestions are only tentative and illustrative. Many other approaches are possible.[37] The important point is to begin to learn on a basis other than the top-down control model of implementation.

References

1 Lomas J and Haynes RB (1987) A taxonomy and critical review of tested strategies for the application of clinical practice recommendations: from official to individual clinical policy. *American Journal of Preventive Medicine,* 4:77.

2 Majone G and Wildavsky A (1979) Implementation as evolution. In: Pressman JL and Wildavsky A., *Implementation: How Great Expectations in Washington are Dashed in Oakland.* University of California Press, Berkeley.

3 Gunn LA (1978) Why is Implementation So Difficult? *Management Services in Government,* 33:169–76.

4 Grimshaw J and Russell IT (1993) Achieving healthy gain through clinical guidelines I: Developing scientifically valid guidelines. *Quality in Health Care,* 2:243–8.

5 Anonymous editorial (1992) *The Lancet,* 339:1197.

6 Kanhouse DE, Winkler JD, Kosecoff J, *et al.* (1989) *Changing Medical Practice Through Technology Assessment.* RAND Corporation, California. p 232.

7 Brook RH and Appell RA (1973) Quality of Care Assessment: choosing a method for peer review. *New Eng Journal Med,* **288:**1323–9.

8 Russell I and Grimshaw J (1992) The effectiveness of referral guidelines: a review of the methods and findings of published evaluations. In: Roland M and Coulter A (eds), *Hospital Referrals.* Oxford University Press, Oxford.

9 Brook RH (1989) Practice guidelines and practicing medicine: are they compatible? *Journal of the American Medical Association,* **262:**3027–30.

10 Mugford M, Banfield P and O'Hanlon M (1991) Effects of feedback of information on clinical practice: a review. *British Medical Journal,* **303:**398–402.

11 Haines A and Feder G (1992) Guidance on guidelines: writing them is easier than making them work. *British Medical Journal,* **305:**785–6.

12 Greco PJ and Eisenberg JM (1993) Changing physicians' practices. *New England Journal of Medicine,* **329:**1271–3.

13 Lipsky M (1980) *Street-Level Bureaucracy.* Russell Sage Foundation, New York.

14 Mintzberg H (1991) The Professional Organization. In: Mintzberg H and Quinn JB (eds), *The Strategy Process: Concepts, Contexts, Cases.* Prentice-Hall, London.

15 Melia KM (1987) *Learning and Working: the Occupational Socialisation of Nurses.* Tavistock, London.

16 Black N and Thompson E (1993) Obstacles to medical audit: British doctors speak. *Social Science and Medicine,* **36:**849–56.

17 Lohr KN and Brook RH (1980) Quality of care in episodes of respiratory illness among Medicaid patients in New Mexico. *Annals of Internal Medicine,* **92:**99–106.

18 Hughes D and Yule B (1991) Incentives and the Remuneration of General Practitioners, *HERU Discussion Paper 02/91.* University of Aberdeen Health Economics Research Unit, Aberdeen.

19 Harrison S and Wistow G (1992) The purchaser/provider split in English health care: towards explicit rationing? *Policy and Politics,* **20:**(2).

20 Brewster CJ, Gill CG and Richbell S (1981) Developing an Analytical Approach to Industrial Relations Policy. *Personnel Review,* **10:**(2).

21 Stocking B (1992) Promoting change in clinical care. *Quality in Health Care,* **1:**56–60.

22 Rogers EM (1983) *The Diffusion of Innovations.* Free Press, New York.

23 Haywood SC and Alaszewski A (1980) *Crisis in the Health Service: the Politics of Management.* Croom Helm, London.
24 Andersen T and Mooney G (eds) (1990) *The Challenge of Medical Practice Variation.* Macmillan, Basingstoke.
25 Lindblom CE (1965) *The Intelligence of Democracy: Decision Making Through Mutual Adjustment.* Free Press, New York.
26 Elmore RF (1979) Backward Mapping: Implementation Research and Policy Decisions. *Political Science Quarterly,* **94**:601–16.
27 Lindblom CE (1959) The Science of Muddling Through. *Public Administration Review,* **19**:79–88.
28 Maas HS (1994) Linking micro and macro in social policy: some historical notes on relevant social science. *Social Policy and Administration,* **28**:174–83.
29 Thompson FJ (1981) *Health Policy and the Bureaucracy.* Massachusetts Institute of Technology Press, London.
30 Tanenbaum SJ (1994) Knowing and acting in Medical Practice: the epistemological politics of outcomes research. *Journal of Health Politics, Policy and Law,* **19**:27–44.
31 Borowitz M and Sheldon TA (1993) Controlling health care: from economic incentives to micro-clinical regulation. *Health Economics,* **2**:201–4.
32 Hunter DJ and Harrison S (1993) *Effective Purchasing for Health Care: Proposals for the first five years.* Report for the NHS Management Executive; University of Leeds Nuffield Institute for Health, Leeds.
33 Allaire Y and Firsirotu ME (1984) Theories of Organizational Culture. *Organization Studies,* **5**.
34 Meek VL (1988) Organizational culture: origins and weaknesses. *Organization Studies,* **9**:453–73.
35 Peters TJ and Waterman RH (1982) *In Search of Excellence.* Harper and Row, New York.
36 Ham CJ, Hunter DJ and Robinson R (1995) Evidence-based policy-making. *British Medical Journal,* **310**:71–2.
37 Harrison S (1994) Knowledge into practice: what's the problem? *Journal of Management in Medicine,* **8**:(2).

11

Future patterns

MARK R BAKER

Illogical logic

Most strategies, and the NHS Research and Development Strategy is no exception, are based on the assumption of a logical progression which leads inexorably towards the desired outcome. For example, legislative change assumes that behaviour change will follow and that the intended outcome will naturally follow. Compulsory seat-belt wearing is an example of this approach being realized whereas the action taken during the mid-1970s to restrict the availability of NHS pay beds led to a perverse and unwanted outcome.

The traditional logical cascade of education, knowledge, attitudes, behaviour and outcome is rarely fulfilled in practice. The R&D strategy relies philosophically on a logical progression of research, knowledge, dissemination, implementation and outcome. There are, however, many twists and uncertainties in this chain which act mainly as obstacles to its success. In general, neither the human nor the organizational elements of the strategy can be regarded as logical; indeed, the strategy itself owes its origins to the apparent absence of a structured approach to government supported health research.

Change, in knowledge-based practice or any other strategic approach, is unpredictable because of the environmental noise created by the absence of anything recognizable as *status quo*, the absence of reliable constants and a superfluity of links in the proposed chain of logical progression. Professional networks can act either as obstacles to the implementation of evidence-based practice (e.g. the fifteen year delay between evidence and the establishment in practice of thrombolytic therapy in acute myocardial infarction) or as stimuli to the widespread adoption of practices which are of unproven benefit (e.g. laparascopic hysterectomy and herniorrhaphy operations).

Soft futures

Traditional planning techniques have been shown to be of limited use in the NHS because of the range and pace of change in clinical practice, service structure and political direction. New approaches to strategy development must enable more flexible and creative responses in an increasingly complex and unstable world. An example of such an approach was the *Future Patterns* project conducted by the author together with the Office for Public Management.[1] This approach used a family of processes known as 'soft futures', which seek to use and build upon the experience and judgement of those involved in real life policy development, and include methods such as the Delphi technique, consensus conferences and behaviour or situation simulations. Through these approaches, and others like them, it is possible to map the vectors and triggers (also known as forces and drivers) for change enabling multi-scenario strategies for the implementation of change to be developed. There are three types of forces acting in direct or indirect ways. At the highest level of abstraction are meta-level forces which are typically beyond the influence of individuals or groups, e.g. demographic change, wealth patterns, wars. At the next level, macro forces operate with a more direct effect on health services; these forces impact through the structure, values and policies which are relevant to health and are within the control of influential groups and lobbies but not of individuals, e.g. fiscal policy on smoking, funding streams in health care, structure of the professions. At the lowest level, micro forces operate at local level, the products of the actions of individuals or groups, e.g. industrial action, development proposals. The three levels of forces are interdependent and they interact, one with another.

The different types and levels of forces operate over different time frames, meta forces operating over the longest term – perhaps extending to years or decades – while micro forces effect change in the short term, days, weeks or months. Of crucial importance to all these forces is the micropolitical context in which they are operating; it is this context which 'soft futures' contends to provide through the wisdom and experience of contemporary change agents.

In the current analysis of the NHS Research and Development Strategy, the main meta level force is the growth of scientific knowledge in health related fields, especially the application of molecular biology techniques to the human genome project. Macro level forces include the research and development strategy itself and the new funding arrangements for research conducted in the NHS which are described elsewhere and are currently being implemented. At the micro level we find a panoply of individual practice changes, each influenced by one or more of the products of the research and development strategy. Thus, we observe a complex mesh of forces and drivers, some competing, others interacting, all contributing to a less than predictable outcome of a unique and ambitious strategy to change the paradigm of health care in the United Kingdom (*see* Box 11.1).

Box 11.1: Levels of forces and drivers and the research and development revolution

Levels	R&D Force/Driver
Meta	Scientific knowledge – global Technology transfer across sectors Human genome project Impact of the cessation of the Cold War on government research and development
Macro	The NHS research and development strategy New funding systems for research and development and for health care The health service research career structure The international Cochrane Collaboration
Micro	Knowledge-based clinical audit Changing individual and group clinical practice Wider involvement in randomized clinical trials Assessing new technologies

---

In a recent future patterns exercise, involving more than fifty experts from clinical, managerial, academic and user backgrounds, the forces and drivers for change were identified from the perspectives of four discrete but overlapping domains, specialist hospital care, priority and community health care, people with continuing health needs and the public and their health. Research-related forces were influential in all these domains but most significantly in specialist hospital care (*see* Box 11.2).

Politics and morality

The apparently universal support for the NHS Research and Development Strategy in high places has surprised many observers. There is no doubt that political patronage across all party lines is an important factor in the success of a strategy whose returns may well span the generations. How

---

Box 11.2: Research and Development forces and drivers in health futures

Service domain	Leading R&D forces and drivers
Specialist hospital care	Increasingly knowledgeable population Skilled utilization of new technologies Extension of (genetic) screening capability New specialties, e.g. genetic therapy/ engineering Better decision-making techniques for purchasers Harmonization of clinical practice (evidence-based)
Primary & community health care	Increasing, knowledge-based, specialization Increasingly knowledgeable population
People with continuing needs	Regulation of research markets Evidence for/against the value of complementary therapies
The public and their health	Universal, research-based, clinical audit Knowledge-based specialization

---

this has been achieved is not altogether clear but it seems likely that the philosophy behind the strategy possesses universal appeal and that there is no obvious process or goal which attracts political opposition.

At the heart of political concerns about health care in developed countries is the need to control the growth in costs without denying access to health care on the grounds of cost. All countries, and all political groups, are troubled by this conundrum and none has yet touched upon a satisfactory answer. It is becoming a widely-held view that rationing health care on cost grounds is a compromise of morality whereas limiting access to health services on the basis of clinical effectiveness enjoys more general support. The apparent support of HM Treasury for the research and development strategy must be based on the alluring prospect of being able to restrict NHS growth by disinvesting from ineffective therapies and procedures. Even at micro level, promoting change management based on research findings is morally superior to any other grounds. It is probably on these principles that political and financial support for the research and development strategy rests. Health services research, unlike molecular biology research and applications, is not important to the health of the wider national economic performance. Therefore, only through the effective delivery of change at local level is governmental support likely to continue.

The functions and manpower review

The review of NHS management structures in 1993 was an inevitable and timely sequel to the reforms of the previous three years. The research and development strategy was merely an appendage to the core changes of the review which were concerned with integrating purchasing and reducing central and regional bureaucracy and management costs. Unfortunately, though predictably, the structures of the fledgling research and development function were swept up in the maelstrom of restructuring and many of the initial leaders and local advocates of the strategy chose to withdraw.

The original decision to base the executive arm of the NHS research and development function in regional health authorities recognized the importance of continuity (RHAs were the only NHS agencies not undergoing reorganization at that time), flexibility (almost all NHS funding rested with RHAs), proximity to the NHS operation/market (RHAs were the market regulators, traditionally the employers of medical staff, the level at which the professions were organized and the line managers of the purchasers) and the need to bring in new people with new ideas, a characteristic for which the NHS is less weak than the Civil Service.

The biphasic implementation of the review, first reducing the number of RHAs from 14 to eight and then absorbing them into the Civil Service, has gone a long way towards eradicating all of the original benefits. It is difficult to see how the gap between the Executive and the NHS can be bridged and it is likely that a more centralized approach to research and development management will strengthen the meta and macro levels but at the expense of weaker influence over the micro setting, where change in practice is effected, the strategy is realized and on which continued political support depends.

Of particular concern is the loss of political, financial and intellectual flexibility which will inevitably result from absorption into the highly politically sensitive, civil service culture. An excessive reliance on logical positivism – belief in the research, knowledge, dissemination, implementation, outcome chain – is unlikely to deliver better health care or improved population health outcomes; it is also likely to fail to deliver the Treasury agenda of reducing overall cost pressures through the selective disinvestment from ineffective measures.

Emerging dilemmas

Few can doubt that the human race sits on the edge of a revolution in its knowledge about itself. The success of the global effort to unlock the secrets of the human genome and its impact on human health and disease is based less on altruism than on the commercial potential of responding to this intellectual property. This, of course, will serve as a stimulus to increase total health service costs, possibly by a factor previously unimagined.

While the continuing development of molecular medicine will progressively expose the mysteries of human susceptibility to disease, and commercial interests lead the drive to invent new ways of responding, the pace of progress in science will probably continue to accelerate. This is not a staggering new insight; the pace of growth of knowledge has continuously accelerated for more than three hundred years; commercial investment in research and development is rising as the potential returns continue to excite. Indeed, an entire new sector of industry has been born to develop science and to convert it to usable technology, that is to solve problems. However, a revolution in health care will lead to an acceleration in the redundancy of the skills of health service staff, including medical practitioners. This will encourage a degree of professional Luddism, challenging the capacity of the health service to deliver change as well as imposing a high human cost as technology eventually triumphs. History suggests that the culture of the NHS workforce is not sufficiently flexible to handle change on this scale. The post-1991 NHS structures and the developing market culture are incompatible with the collective approaches which have characterized most changes in professional practice notwith-standing the inherently competitive nature of some professions. This is not necessarily an indictment of the new arrangements but we have not yet learnt how to predict with any accuracy the outcome of the various forces operating in the NHS market. Furthermore, the loss of the regional tier of management has deprived the service of both its safety net and most of its flexibility. Innovation in health services research will prove to be one of the victims.

The future for the NHS research and development strategy

Four important macro level forces are currently conspiring against the continuing success of the research and development strategy (Box 11.3). Two of these concern the structure of the research community; the other two concern NHS structure and culture. First, the research community undervalues health services research – relative to other health research –

and the national research capacity is insufficient to meet the growing requirements of the NHS and the expectations of the Treasury. Second, this undervaluation, characterized by the low value placed on applied research in the higher education research selectivity exercise, is reflected in the absence of any discernible career structure for health service researchers in the country. Third, this situation is further exacerbated by the centralization of power in the NHS Executive which, based on the previous record of the Department of Health, suggests that neither of the research infrastructure problems is likely to be adequately addressed. Finally, the successful implementation of evidence-based practice requires the knowledge culture to be internalized into the delivery of health care. This involves not just providers of care but also the purchasers who, in a mature market, will dictate the rules. The purchasing framework is itself fragmented between health authorities, GP fundholders and primary care total purchasing schemes. While it is by no means clear that health authority leadership will prove to be effective in achieving evidence-based health care, it is generally accepted that primary care-led purchasing is less likely to espouse and effectively promote research-based practice. As has proved the case with many of the changes since 1991, the general practitioners may yet surprise us. Being macro level forces, these four factors ought to be the target of co-ordinated management action.

Box 11.3: The macro forces of opposition

- Applied research, and health services research in particular, is undervalued by the higher education and research community; this is reflected in the lower value given to applied research in the universities' research selectivity exercise.

- There is no formal, or recognizable informal, career structure for health service researchers. There are few senior research posts and most staff, even at senior level, do not enjoy tenure.

- The Department of Health, in the form of the NHS Executive, now possesses control over policy and funding of NHS research. It was the continuing failure of this Department to adequately address the above issues, amongst others, that led to the development of the R&D strategy in the first place.

- The loss of collectivism, the fragmentation of the health purchasing role and the lack of relevant skills and vision in DHA's conspire against effective implementation of research-based practice at local level.

Basic sociological principles suggest that success depends on the acceptance of responsibility for changing practices by the key professions themselves, hence the glimmer of hope for the primary care leadership role. The post-industrial world has not yet come to terms with the replacement of job security through employment by security through the possession of relevant and valued skills. The health professions may come to realize that their most powerful asset of statutory self-determination and self-government may only survive if they embrace the vital attributes of flexibility and responsiveness to evidence. If this path is followed, and medicine is perhaps the profession most likely to, not only will the cemeteries be overflowing with sacred cows but users of health services may even enjoy better and more predictable outcomes.

References

1 Office for Public Management (1995) *Future Patterns*. London.

Index

applicability *see* development of results
applied research
  low value of 121
  versus pure research 42
asthma 86
audit 106–7
  influencing results 108

Bandolier (newsletter) 35
Berkowitz, David 28
Bornholm's epidemic myalgia 76
British Medical Journal (BMJ) 27–8, 33

care in the community 39
Central Research and Development
    Committee (CRDC) 7, 31, 38, 84–5
Centre for Reviews and Dissemination
    (CRD) 32–3, 35, 44, 81
cervical screening 86, 107
chairs (professor posts) 46, 70
Clearing House on Health Outcomes 36
clinical trials 12–15
  anonymity and confidentiality 14–15
  informed consent 10, 12–13
  meta-analysis 15, 21
  patient selection 11
  randomized controlled model 55–7
  termination of 15
  types of 13, 16, 55–6
clinicians
  enthusiasm for innovation 25–6
  goals of 25
  information overload and 27–8

research priorities 22–3
Cochrane Centres 32, 36, 44, 81
Cochrane Collaboration 20, 32, 44
collaborative nature of health care 108–9
collaborative research 42–4
commissioning research 91–3
communications systems 24–5
community-based R&D 46
computerization *see* information
    technology
consensus conference 20
contract researchers 41–2
costs *see* funding of research
cot deaths 77
CRD 32–3, 35, 44, 81
CRDC 7, 31, 38, 84–5
Culyer Report (1994) 6, 37–49, 84

development of results 31–4, 103–14
  application gap 61
  bottom-up implementation 109–10
  ethical issues 12
  information overload 27–8
  strategic model 110–11
  top-down implementation 104–9
diabetes 86
dissemination *see* development of
    results
doctors *see* clinicians; GPs

Effective Health Care Bulletins 30, 32, 35
  Pregnancy and Childbirth 33
epidemiological research 43, 52

Essential National Health Research (WHO concept) 51
ethical issues 9–18
  clinical trials 12–15
  ethics committees 6, 10, 14
  Health Systems Research 55
Evans Commission 51
Evidence-Based Purchasing (digest) 35
  Bandolier (newsletter) 35

financial incentives 86, 107–8
funding of research 24, 38–40, 97–8
  commissioning research 91–3
  England total R&D funding 45
  funding management 97–8
  for nurses and PAMs 67–8
  political aspects 118
  underfunding complaints 38
Future Patterns project 116

general practice/primary care settings 75–86
GPs 46, 121–2
  drug companies and 28
  referral rates 76, 79
  university GP/primary care departments 76
  guidelines *see* development of results

Health Advisory Service 112
health authorities 46–7
health purchasers *see* purchasers
health research, *definition* 51–2
Health Services Journal 28
health services research 51–62
  undervalued 120–1
Health Systems Research (WHO concept) 51, 54
Health Technology Assessment programme 7
human genome project 116, 120
Hungin, Pali 83

IFM Healthcare 35
immunization, target payments and 86, 107

implementation *see* development of results
incentives (financial) 86, 107–8
infectious hepatitis 76
information technology (IT)
  data overload and 24–5
  general practice computerization 79, 85
  information systems strategy 31–3
  investments in 28–9
  on-line patient-specific reminders 106
  priority setting 30
Integrated Clinical Work Stations (ICWS) 27
Internet 24, 27

journals 27–8, 106

librarians 29, 35

managers
  goals of 25
  influencing clinical behaviour 107
  information overload and 28
  research priorities 22–3
  research project management 93–102
  research skills needed 45, 54
managing research and development 89–102
  commissioning research 91–3
  project management 93–102
medical audit 106–7
  influencing results 108
medical journals 27–8, 106
Medical Research Council (MRC) 1
Medline 29
Mental Health programme 7
molecular medicine 116, 120
MRC (Medical Research Council) 1
myocardial infarction 92–3, 115

National Forum 38, 41
National Morbidity Surveys 76
National Research Register 32, 35, 44
NHS Executive Regional Offices 6
n-of-1 trial 16
Northern Research Network 83–4

Nuremberg code 13–14
nurses 106, 108
nursing research 65–73
Nursing Times 28

Oral Contraceptive Study 76
out-reach clinics 79

paramedical professions 65–73
patients' charter 78
Peckham, Michael 2–3, 31
personal chairs 46, 70
pilot studies 96–7
placebo effect 19
politics and morality 118
    research priorities 22
pressure sore prevention/management
    68
primary care settings 72, 75–86
Priorities in Medical Research (1988) 1–2
professions allied to medicine (PAMs)
    65–73
professorships 46, 70
Project Registers System 32, 35, 44
promotion procedures for research staff
    41
protocol development 54–5
purchasers 46–7
    goals of 25
    NHS purchasing and GP
        fundholding 78
    research funding and 84
    research priorities 22–3
Purchasing Innovations Database 36
pure *v* applied research 42

qualitative approaches 58–61

referral rates of GPs 76, 79
Regional and Central R&D Committee
    (CRDC) 7, 31, 38, 84–5
Regional Health Authorities (RHAs) 6,
    66, 119
Regional Offices (ROs) 6

Research for Health (1991) 4–5, 31
Research for Health (1993) 31, 33, 83
research workers
    absence of career structure 121
    needs of 41–2
Resource Management Initiative (RMI)
    27
review of NHS management structures
    119
Royal College of General Practitioners
    76, 84

senior lectureships 46
senior registrar posts 76
Service Increment for Teaching and
    Research (SIFTR) 39, 41, 68, 84
*Strategy for Research in Nursing, Midwifery
    and Health Visiting* (1992) 65
study designs 13, 16
    see also clinical trials
support units for research 96
survey research methods 57–8

Taking Research Seriously (1990) 2
Task Force on R&D in the NHS 37–48,
    65, 68
teamwork *see* collaborative
training in research for GPs 83
trusts
    research strategies 45–6, 68–70
    SIFTR and 68
    University Chairs in Nursing and 70

unemployment, health consequences 76
universities
    GP/primary care departments 76
    research selectivity exercise 121
    SIFTR and 41
    university chairs 46, 70
    university-linked medical posts 1

vaccination, target payments for 86, 107

Zelen protocols 12–13